WINDOW OF THE SOUL:

A Brief Exploration of the Human Eye

David Baker

Published in 2018 by FeedARead.com Publishing

A CIP catalogue record for this title is available from the British Library.

The eye is the jewel of the body.'

Henry David Thoreau

'Who are you going to believe, me or your own eyes?'

Groucho Marx

For Julie, Avi, Daniel and my mother.

In remembrance of my father, who showed me that being an optometrist is, first and foremost, about people.

CONTENTS

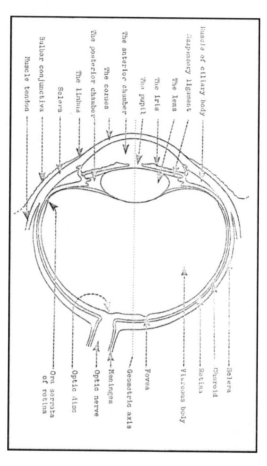

Figure 1. Horizontal cross-section of the human eye.

8

INTRODUCTION

'The Creature has a purpose and his eyes are bright with it.' John Keats

The complexity of the human eye has often been used as an example to illustrate the argument for creation. How can it be possible, the anti-evolutionist line goes, for such an incredible structure to come about purely by chance and natural selection? However the eye got to where it is today, it *is* an incredible feat of bioengineering, albeit with some seemingly illogical design features built in.

A reading chart that I use in my work as an optometrist starts with the words, 'The eye can be strikingly compared with a camera which is in constant use from morning to night...' Well, up to a point. More striking are the differences; the amazing versatility and sensitivity of the eye when compared with a camera, a camcorder or, for that matter, any other man-made imaging instrument.

The various organs of the human body are necessarily unique in their own ways because of the particular functions which they are designed to perform. The eye has a special place, however, in the story of the human body. It provides our primary source of information about the outside world, both spatial (in three dimensions when both eyes are used together) and temporal, allowing us to know how our environment changes with time. The eyes are the key to a person's expressions, moods and inner feelings, thus facilitating sophisticated social interactions. Perhaps in proportion to the quantity of information they receive, so is the amount of information which they convey.

When I started out as an optometry undergraduate at Aston University, in Birmingham, back in 1983, the anatomy lecturer at the time began the Ocular Anatomy course with a statement which hints at the fascinating nature of the visual sense organ, concisely and almost poetically:

'The eye - a small, delicate, beautifully intricate organ comprising a greater diversity of tissues than any other single part of the body.'

One could add (take a deep breath): the eye - a globe of diameter two and a half centimetres, weighing a mere seven grams, with approximately 137 million light-sensitive cells which turn light into electrical signals to be sent along a million nerve fibres comprising the optic nerve; half of these fibres, on their journey through the brain, cross over at a junction with the other optic nerve in a dazzlingly complex but precise, ordered, fashion to the opposite pathway, reaching the visual processing centre, or cortex, at the back of the brain; culminating in the production of an intelligible, upright, three-dimensional, stable, colour picture - the end result of two slightly different upside-down images formed on the retinas of two eyes, about six centimetres apart, in a constantly moving head.

This stable image is formed, despite constant head and eye movements, despite constantly blinking eyelids obstructing the view and despite changing levels of illumination tens of times greater than anything the best cameras can cope with. There is a variable aperture to control light entering the eye and to adjust depth of focus, a system to permit almost instantaneous change of focus for almost any distance and a system of six muscles attached to each eye, working in pairs and in concert with the muscles of the opposite eye, all of which helps to maintain the clear three-dimensional picture whether the eyes are moving in the same direction (say, tracking an object moving across the field of vision) or in opposite directions (say, watching an object move closer).

And one might mention in passing that when you see someone wearing *really* thick spectacles, the lenses might have a strength of 10 dioptres (dioptres being the units of optical focusing power); exceptionally, even 20 dioptres. The eye's own optical system has a power of almost 60 dioptres, with a capacity (diminishing with age) to increase by another 15 - 20 dioptres when required.

And - breathe out! I think I prefer my lecturer's summary, but there in a rather large nutshell is some of what makes the eye so fascinating. It is no wonder then, that the eye and the mechanics of vision have exercised some of the greatest scientific minds throughout history.

In unravelling the some of the mysteries of vision, we will encounter no fewer than four Lucasian Professors, the Cambridge University post held by the late Stephen Hawking. We will encounter an Astronomer Royal; find a connection between the founding of Pennsylvania, the understanding of colour vision and the inventor of calculators; and meet the decoder of the Rosetta Stone. We will also pay homage to some of the pioneering anatomists and physiologists who teased out the minute structure and workings of the eye. Which is not even to mention the strange case of Leonardo da Vinci, René Descartes and the invention of contact lenses...

Let me take you on a journey of exploration to celebrate these human sense organs for the detection of electromagnetic radiation between the infra-red and ultraviolet wavelengths. Along the way we will peer into the Canal of Schlemm and marvel at the Zonules of Zinn. It may take your breath away; or at least it might answer some of those questions that you've been itching to ask as you sat in the optometrist's consulting room chair (like – 'what exactly *is* an optometrist, anyway: I always see the optician?').

By the end of the journey you may never see (or look at) things in quite the same way. What follows is not intended to be a text book of ocular anatomy or physiology. In fact, some parts of the eye are only very briefly sketched out. I have concentrated on what I consider to be the most fascinating aspects; the aspects which I most frequently get asked about, and the aspects that are so amazing most people don't even know about. I will keep units of measurement as simple as possible: apart from commonly used kilometres (km), metres (m), centimetres (cm) and millimetres (mm), I will use micrometres (μm), which are 0.000001m, to describe microscopic dimensions; and microlitres (μl), which are 0.000001 litres, for volume. It could be argued that nanometres (nm), 0.000000001 metres, should be used as well, since wavelengths of light and dimensions of microscopic structures of the eye are often stated in these units, but I have elected to stick with micrometres for ease of comparison of size of all the small items described.

This tour through the eye is intended to give a flavour of how the eye works; or, given its strange construction, should that be: 'how on earth does the eye work?'

CHAPTER ONE

THE BIRTH OF SIGHT

'The eyes are the window of the soul.' Proverbs

Look into your partner's eyes; go on - gaze deeply into them. Or, if your partner is not to hand, or you have no partner, make eye contact with the person sitting opposite you on the train, or ...well, you get the drift. The point is, that when you look at someone's eyes, you are looking at their brain. Not in the sense of knowing their mind by the eyes' expression, although that is certainly an important psychological effect; I mean the fact that the eyes are not only made of the same stuff as the brain, they are direct outgrowths of it.

The development of the eyes from the embryonic brain material, and the wealth of connections between these organs, as well as the proportion of the brain devoted to the sense of sight, reflect the importance of vision to our understanding of the world about us. Consider the fact that as much as half of the brain's cerebral cortex is concerned with visual function, whether directly in perception or, through complex interconnections, for the interpretation and understanding of visual information. Consider also, that of the twelve so-called cranial nerves, those nerves that originate in the brain, five, i.e. nearly half, are concerned with the eye in some way.

General Development

Before plunging into the intricacies of ocular development, it is worth pausing to consider the framework within which the human embryo as a whole grows. This will provide a context in which to look at the growth of the eyes. Once the mother's egg has been fertilised by a single sperm, there are certain landmarks in the development of the embryo and foetus that are worth noting, which may be interesting to refer back to when following the timetable of growth of the eye.

Early on in the embryonic stage, during the third week of growth, the cardiovascular system begins to form. Pools of blood appear which are lined by cells that become the basis of vessel walls. These pools become arranged in isolated clusters which fuse, giving rise to blood vessels. By the fourth week a single, primitive heart tube is formed, with eventually two heart tubes appearing. In the third month the heart begins to beat - a process which continues uninterrupted (hopefully) around 70 times per minute for in the region of 70 – 90 years.

The first signs of arms and legs appear as fore- and hind-limb buds at around five weeks, although most of the growth of the limbs occurs later on. The fourth month is characterised by the onset of formation of the skeleton.

During the fifth month the foetus will begin to start moving its extremities, with a force which most mothers will readily be able to describe.

At around seven weeks, the sex organs start to become differentiated; before this the embryo is potentially of either sex developmentally. The stimulus to growth of the relevant organs (which at the same time results in the regression of the opposite sex organs) is from the Y chromosome in the male, and from the XX chromosome combination in the female.

The foetal period, starting at around nine weeks, is characterised by a large spurt in growth of the body, now that the body parts are largely defined. An illustration of this increase in the rate of growth is that, at two months, the head makes up 50 per cent of 'crown-rump' (CR) length (ie head-to-bottom), whereas at birth, the ratio is reduced to 20 per cent of CR. In other words, there is an explosion of growth of the body during this period with respect to growth of the head.

This, then, is a very brief outline of the process which has produced you and me, much like a time-lapse film which reduces hours of observation to a few minutes of running time. Now we will home in on the aspects of prenatal development which concern the eyes.

Ocular Development

In describing the events comprising the development of the eye, I will mention various parts of the eye whose functions will be explained in subsequent chapters. So as not to interrupt the flow of narrative of the following unfolding sequence of events, I will not at this stage digress with too many anatomical definitions. All should become clear in subsequent chapters. The important thing is to be able to appreciate a sense of the evolution of the developmental process.

The optical story begins, essentially, at only 25 days when a structure called the optic primordium becomes visible as an outward-folding projection of the outer walls of the most primitive neural tissue structure, the neural tube.

Now, the three primary brain vesicles, or cavities, develop; the optic primordia grow into bulbs connected with the forebrain by stalks. We have reached 28 days. The optic bulbs make contact with another embryonic cell tissue type, which is stimulated by this contact to begin developing the embryonic lens of the eye.

This is part of a pre-determined, orderly sequence of tissue interactions, where each stage stimulates the onset of a succeeding stage. One occasionally sees a child with a partial or complete absence of one of the structures of the eye. The severity of the defect depends upon when the onset of the abnormal development takes place; the earlier the onset, the more profound is the structural defect. It is partly because of the strict sequential nature of pre-natal development that children with birth, or congenital, ocular defects, often have defects of other parts of the body, as part of a wider syndrome. It is almost a wonder that the delicately choreographed sequence of events which result in a healthy baby is not upset more often than it is.

To return to our timetable: the lens is beginning its development. This induces the optic bulb to invaginate, or fold inwards, forming a double-walled optic cup, by 32 days. The optic cup grows in such a way as to leave a fissure at the base of the cup into which a branch of the carotid artery grows. This small branch, the hyaloid artery, carries in cells which, it is believed, form part of the vitreous body.

Fast-forward to five weeks. Pigment appears in cells of the outer wall of the optic cup, while the thicker inner wall begins to form the neural retina, the tissue which eventually contains nerve cells connected, via the optic nerve, to the brain.

After a further two weeks, i.e. seven weeks in total, the surface of the cornea (the epithelium) has become a well-defined layer two cells deep. This growth is another step triggered by the embryonic lens. Meanwhile, the other layers of the cornea are beginning to develop. Around this time, there is also some development of eyelid folds and extra-ocular muscles (the muscles that move the eyes).

At eight and a half weeks the iris starts to form, and the lens becomes enveloped in a membrane - the lens capsule. The capsule is significant for cataract operations, where the lens itself is removed - of which more later. It is around this time that the retinal neural cells, referred to previously, will have developed; and will have grown long bodies, or axons, which leave in the cavity of the stalk connecting the eye to the brain. These long fibres collectively become the optic nerve.

Let us pause for a moment, at the threshold of the final, 'foetal stage' of growth. We have seen how the eyes develop from proto-brain material, and we have reached the point where most of the different structures of the eye have been delineated, and the optic nerve has established communication lines with the brain. It is a little like the erection of a new building, where the framework has been completed and is ready for the installation of the infra-structure. All this, and the foetus is still only about 26mm from head to bottom. So now we round off pre-natal ocular development with a rollercoaster ride through the foetal stage.

- Three months: the eyelids have fused together; the muscles of the eyelids and the muscles which dilate and constrict the pupil are forming.

- Four months: the structure of the cornea is nearly complete. The ciliary body (which produces aqueous fluid), the ciliary muscle (which controls lens focusing) and the canal of Schlemm (which drains away aqueous fluid) are all under construction.

- Six months: the extra-ocular muscles become attached to the outer coating of the eye, the sclera. There is more eyelid development with the formation of glands, eyelashes and the conjunctiva, which lines the inner surface of the lids.

- Seven months: the diameter of the eyeball is in the region of 10-14mm. The optic nerve begins to be covered with a fatty myelin sheath, which helps to maintain the speedy conduction of nerve signals along it. Some multiple sclerosis sufferers have symptoms of visual disturbances, which is due to deterioration of this coating.

- Nine months: the eye's diameter is 16-17mm. The retina is almost fully formed, and myelination of the optic nerve is complete. The remains of the hyaloid artery, having completed its task, can be seen at its two ends: at the optic disc, where it and the optic nerve enter the eye; and on the rear surface of the lens. These remnants can even be observed in some adults. The empty length of the artery may be seen in the vitreous body as a structure called the canal of Cloquet. Until now, the iris has been covered by a membrane. This now disintegrates, leaving a gap in the circular central section which is the pupil, and resulting in an undulating front surface of the iris which is what we see as the iris pattern, unique to the individual. In white races, the iris will not have acquired pigment at this time; so white babies generally have blue eyes.

Post-natal Ocular Development

The eye, as with many other organs, does not spring forth with the baby from the womb in a fully mature state. Birth does not provide a full-stop, merely a series of commas indicating a gradual evolution. There is also an inexorable degeneration, from the moment of formation of a structure, until death. The lens is unique in the eye in that it alone continues to grow progressively throughout life.

During the first four months after birth, the central or, macular, region of the retina undergoes cellular organisation. The macula is the most sensitive part of the retina, which is responsible for most of the detail of the image formed by the eye. This is also the period within which the upper visual pathways (from the rear end of the optic nerve towards the visual cortex of the brain) become myelinated.

How visually aware are babies of their surroundings at this early age? A weak reflex, sufficient for a baby to fix on to an object briefly, may be present at birth. By between five and six weeks a reflex linking the eyes is developed enough to allow the eyes to follow a light. At seven or eight weeks the blink reflex appears, and by three months the eyes will track an object, thus marking a transition from reflex to conscious fixation on objects. A series of changes can be noted at around six months, such as the ability of the eyes to coordinate their movements in a more refined way, and the development of pigment which causes a change in iris colour.

Vision in Babies

Let's first deal with the obvious question: how does one measure a baby's eyesight? Not by sitting the few-months-old baby in a chair whilst asking it questions and getting it to read a letter chart, that's for sure. One method relies on the fact that, given two objects to look at, the baby will tend to look at a detailed, moving picture in preference to a static, plain one. Once the interesting, moving object is reduced to a size where a preference is no longer demonstrable, it can be concluded that the limit of the baby's vision has been reached. Not unreasonably, this is called the 'preferential looking' technique. These tests are often performed by orthoptists (see Appendix A) in a hospital eye department.

The vision of a newborn baby is approximately equivalent to being able to see a letter twice as large as the largest letter on a normal eye test chart. Interestingly, this translates roughly to baby being able to make out mother's face when being held in her arms. Within the first five to seven years of life the vision improves to the adult level of 20/20 (as the Americans say), or 6/6 (as we say in the UK - because we measure testing distances in metres, the Americans in feet: see Appendix B).

In these early days there is simultaneous development of other parts of the visual system such as: the ability to adjust focus, the facility of depth perception and the greater control of a range of eye movements. However, the visual system actually starts to form *in utero*, before any visual experience is possible. Studies of newborn macaque monkeys have shown that some cells found in the adult monkey are already present. Electrical activity in the cells of the foetus plays a vital role in the development of normal anatomical connections in the visual system; it has been found that, in mammalian foetal retinas, cells fire large electrical signals even though there is no visual stimulus. Blockage of these signals by chemical means prevents normal development of the visual cortex.

At this point, turn away if you do not like animal experiments. There is a post-natal critical period for visual development, and experiments by such researchers as David Hubel and Torsten Wiesel - famous in their field - mainly on cats and monkeys, have revealed much information about this time, which is of vital importance for the treatment of young children's visual problems.

Hubel, who died in 2013, and Wiesel found that suturing closed a newborn monkey's eyes resulted in profound blindness when the eyelids were opened some days later. An adult monkey deprived of a visual image (not unlike a human with cataracts) suffers no loss of visual function once the blockage or deprivation is removed.

Suturing closed one eye of a monkey during the critical period even for a short time deprives that eye of the ability to influence visual cortex cells to react to stimuli. But this effect can be corrected by opening that eye and suturing closed the other eye.

This critical period, then, corresponds to a time when the wiring in the visual cortex of the brain is still developing and is therefore capable of being shaped. It really is striking that depriving the retina of visual stimulation produces anomalies of connections in the visual cortex; in other words, sensory deprivation alone alters the anatomy of this part of the brain. Note that no physical harm is done to the eye itself by any such deprivation.

That visual sensory deprivation alone will cause abnormalities in the anatomical wiring of the visual cortex would suggest that other areas of the cerebral cortex completely unrelated to vision may also require adequate sensory stimulation during a critical period, in order to form sufficient anatomical connections for normal adult functioning. Provision of a varied and interesting sensory environment for babies and young children would, therefore, seem to be of vital importance to their development.

Certainly, the Hubel and Wiesel research has profound clinical implications for the treatment of paediatric eye problems. It suggests that the early removal of congenital cataract, and detection of refractive errors such as myopia (short-sight), hypermetropia (long-sight) and astigmatism (see Chapter Three) and their correction with spectacles are extremely important; as is the early correction of squints (one eye turns in or out), so that the cortical pathways concerning binocular vision can form within the critical period. The critical period in humans covers around the first seven years, so any treatment must be performed as early as possible within this time so as to achieve the best results.

We are now able to arrive at a better understanding of the familiar term 'lazy eye'. The eye itself is healthy and works perfectly well. It sends off its signals up the optic nerve to the visual cortex, but the wiring is not developed enough to be able to interpret the signals. Spectacles alone make no difference, since the problem lies in the brain, not the eye. If this situation becomes ingrained within the critical period, the brain adjusts to allow suppression of the resultant fuzzy image produced by the poor processing of the signals sent by the retina (which may have a beautifully sharp, focused, image formed on it). The suppression enables the clear image produced by the other eye and its associated cortical area to be highlighted.

This is why young children are sometimes to be seen wearing a patch over one eye. The eye being covered is actually the good eye. This hopefully ensures the weak eye is stimulated sufficiently for the cortical development to take place, thus avoiding suppression and the consequent 'lazy eye'. It used to be thought that patching throughout the day, or at least for several hours a day, was required to produce the necessary improvement in the weak eye; but

26

concerns arose regarding the health of the good eye if it was covered for such long periods during the critical phase of visual development.

In any case it was – and is, as any parent will tell you – very difficult to get a child to wear a patch at all, let alone in public. Not only would the child be terribly self-conscious about it and be liable to teasing by its peers, but there is the inescapable logic, from the child's point of view, of: remove the patch and see better!

The type of patching regime more commonly used now is to cover the good eye for an hour or two per day at home, during which period the child is encouraged to perform detailed tasks such as reading or colouring-in as neatly as possible, or even playing computer games. Yes – according to recent research computer games can (or perhaps one should say cautiously, *might be*) good for vision in certain circumstances.

In summary, we have seen that the eyes are indeed outposts of the brain - on stalks - and that information passed along those stalks (the optic nerves) during a critical period of childhood is vital to the development of a properly functioning visual system. In the next chapters we will delve deeper into the wondrous structures of the eye to find out how the organ of sight gathers the necessary information. Our journey will begin at the front of the eye and take us more or less in a straight line to the back – and beyond.

CHAPTER TWO

THE CONJUNCTIVA

'The hardest thing to see is what is in front of your eyes.'
Johann Wolfgang von Goethe

The conjunctiva is well known as the part of the eye that is responsible for that group of annoying conditions that gives rise to red, sore, itchy, watery and sticky eyes. In many cases the minor infection responsible will gradually peter out over about a week if left alone, or seven days if treated with antibacterial eyedrops. The conjunctiva also provides the answer to the perennial question asked of contact lens practitioners: 'Can my contact lens get stuck round the back of my eye?'

But what and where exactly is the conjunctiva? It is thanks largely to a father and son pair of anatomists that we can say more than that it is just vaguely somewhere at the front of the eye. And the work of a French surgeon, a member of an academy whose members included Napoleon Bonaparte, gave the first detailed description of the relationship between the conjunctiva and the eyeball itself.

Professor of anatomy at Hanover, Carl Friedrich Theodore Krause (1797 – 1868) made extensive studies of the dimensions of the human eye and is remembered by the conjunctival glands of Krause. Not to be outdone, his son, Wilhelm (1833 – 1910), was professor of pathological anatomy at Göttingen University for thirty-one years, afterwards working at the Anatomical Institute in Berlin. He also made huge contributions to ocular anatomy, researching the refractive index of various parts of the eye, the structure of the retina and the nerve supply of the cornea and conjunctiva. While working on the anatomy of the muscles and sensory nerves of the body, he described nerve-endings in the conjunctiva and other tissues now known as the 'end-bulbs of Krause'. The Krauses laid the foundations for the description of the conjunctiva that follows.

There are four distinct regions of the conjunctiva:

1. *Palpebral conjunctiva* - which is subdivided into *marginal, tarsal* and *orbital* regions.

2. *Fornix* - which is subdivided into *superior, inferior, lateral* and *medial* regions.

3. *Bulbar conjunctiva* - which is subdivided into *scleral* and *limbal* regions.

4. *Plica semilunaris.*

Starting at the edge of the eyelids, the palpebral conjunctiva is directly continuous with the skin of the outer surface of the lids. This is the marginal zone, which extends a short way up the inside surface of the lids, until it merges with the tarsal region. At this point, there is a small groove called the *subtarsal sulcus* running parallel to the lid margin. It is an ideal place for annoying little foreign bodies to lodge in. The tarsal conjunctiva contains many small blood vessels and, unlike the marginal and orbital portions of the palpebral conjunctiva, is tightly and immovably fixed to the underlying lid.

That Contact Lens Question

From the orbital conjunctiva, covering the upper part of the inside of the lids, we move to the fornix. The word 'fornix' derives from the Latin for arch, or vault, which describes the shape of the structure. Incidentally, the word 'fornication' comes from the same Latin root; Roman prostitutes often solicited from under the arches of particular buildings. The fornix is a fold of conjunctival tissue that goes from around from the top of the inside lid surface to the surface of the eyeball, thereby making an outer lining for a mucous membrane that follows the same path.

The important thing to realise is that this anatomical arrangement forms a cul-de-sac; if one could travel along the space between the lids and the eyeball, one would reach a dead end. The fornix creates a physical barrier to the back of the eyeball. An errant contact lens - or anything else, for that matter - just cannot get past the fornix. Actually, very, very rarely, it *can* happen; but that's just the extremely unlikely exception that proves the rule. So it's worth emphasising the point, because it's such a com-

31

mon fear: that for all intents and purposes, *a contact lens cannot go behind the eye*.

The seal formed by the fornix runs all the way round the inside furthest extent of the eyelids where they meet the eyeball, from the nasal limit of the upper lid to the nasal limit of the lower lid via the temporal (outer) limit of the lids where they meet. Hence we have the *superior, lateral* and *inferior* fornix. At the nasal corner of the eye where the lids meet, there is a different anatomical arrangement for the *medial* fornix.

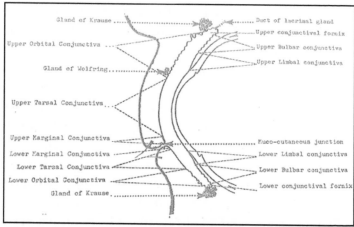

Figure 2. Vertical cross-section of eyelids (and front of eye) showing the segments of conjunctiva.

A look in the mirror reveals a knobbly, roughly triangular, area right in the nasal corner of the eye by the meeting of the lids. This structure is called the *caruncle*. It contains two types of sebaceous glands, each with its own specific function. One type contributes secretions to the oily layer of the tears (see Chapter Four). The other glands' secretions lubricate, soften and coat foreign bodies that become deposited on the caruncle during the action of blinking. These latter glands are found surrounding each of the many 1mm-long hairs that cover the caruncle, which themselves have the job of trapping debris and foreign bodies. The under-surface of the caruncle is connected to one of the external muscles that moves the eyeball (the medial rectus), so that it moves slightly when the eye is turned left or right.

Look even closer in the mirror and immediately adjacent to the caruncle is a crescent-shaped structure which is a fold of conjunctival tissue called the *plica semilunaris*. The medial fornix contains the caruncle and plica. Some animals have a full or partial third eyelid, or nictitating membrane, which provides extra protection and moisture while maintaining vision. The human eye does not have such a membrane, but the fact that smooth muscle fibres are occasionally found in the plica hints at a distant connection. The folded tissue of the plica acts as a mechanism for allowing sufficient movement of the lids and eyeball, and also the maintenance of good drainage of the tear film. As the eye moves left or right, the plica folds or unfolds to enable smooth movement of the eyeball.

The thinnest part of the conjunctiva is that which continues from the fornix, across the white of the eye (sclera) to the edge of the cornea (the subject of the next chapter), where the superficial (epithelial) layer becomes continuous with the corneal epithelium as the deeper layers of the conjunctiva end. This is the bulbar conjunctiva. The junction of the cornea and sclera is called the *limbus*, hence the division of bulbar conjunctiva into scleral and limbal portions.

That Looks Serious!

The bulbar conjunctiva, as just mentioned, is very thin. So thin, in fact, that its transparency allows the blood vessels beneath to be easily seen. When some of these vessels become dilated, the appearance created is what we call a 'red eye'. Eye whitening eyedrops work by constricting these vessels so that they become less visible, making the eye appear whiter. But blood vessels carry, among other things, oxygen to tissues and, if such drops are used too frequently, those tissues start sending signals as if to say, 'Hang on, we're not getting enough oxygen here!' so extra blood is pumped their way. This results in a type of redness of the eye called 'rebound hyperaemia'; in other words, overuse of eye whitening drops can actually lead to a redder eye.

There are many causes of red eye, such as haemorrhage, infection, allergy and inflammation. One of these is the *subconjunctival haemorrhage*. This is a very common, but very dramatic-looking variety of red eye. As its name suggests, the condition's appearance is due to a leakage of blood into the space beneath the conjunctiva, overlying the white of the eye, the sclera. The blood is a result of a rupture of one of the small adjacent blood vessels. But it is almost invariably painless, so the first anyone knows about it is either when someone says, 'Good grief! Have you seen your eye? What have you done to it?' Or maybe looking in a mirror provides the initial shock of seeing a solid block of brick-red on the white of the eye.

It certainly looks serious but, fortunately, it almost always isn't; and because its appearance is so distinctive, it is usually very easy for the optometrist or doctor to diagnose it. In the majority of cases, it is a one-off chance occurrence, often with an unknown cause (idiopathic); or it may happen as a result of a so-called valsalva manoeuvre such as a violent cough or sneeze that creates enough temporary pressure from the neck up to 'pop' one of the small, delicate vessels in or around the conjunctiva. But repeated subconjunctival haemorrhage might indicate that the blood pressure is raised on a more long-term basis, and the doctor or optometrist should take a careful history of the patient to exclude rarer causes such as head trauma, certain systemic diseases and medicinal side-effects.

Diseases of the conjunctiva account for a large proportion of those conditions referred to as 'red eye'. Most people have had a red eye at one time or another, and there is a whole host of possible causes. The term *conjunctivitis* applies to an inflammation of the conjunctiva, usually with associated reddening of the eye. The most common causes are infections, allergies and irritants. Infections can be bacterial, viral and fungal and of varying severity and seriousness. Allergies may be seasonal (eg pollen) or perennial (eg dust mites). They may be acquired after repeated exposure to particular ingredients in such things as eyedrops and make-up. Sometimes repeated mechanical rubbing of a contact lens can induce a particular type of allergic conjunctivitis in a previously happy lens wearer. Finally, airborne or waterborne chemical irritants that the eye comes into contact with can result in conjunctivitis.

We have now completed a fairly detailed tour of the conjunctiva, but what of our French surgeon and colleague of Napoleon who was mentioned at the beginning of the chapter? Actually, he is not directly associated with the conjunctiva itself, but the anatomical feature named after him is intimately related to it and not only has a bearing on the way the eye is able to move freely but is crucial to modern eye surgical techniques.

Jacques René Tenon (1724 – 1826) was a noted anatomist, surgeon and ophthalmologist in Paris, who became surgeon-in-chief of the Salpêtrière hospital, built at the instigation of Louis XIV on the site of a gunpowder factory (hence its name). By 1789 it was the largest hospital in the world, catering for up to ten thousand patients. He also became a member of the Institute of France, first class. The Institute, founded in 1795 by the French Revolutionary

Government, was in part an amalgamation of other long-standing prestigious academies and societies. Tenon, along with Napoleon Bonaparte, was one of its earliest members.

As part of his anatomical studies Tenon described a fine layer of fibro-elastic tissue covering virtually the whole of the eyeball. Who cared? Pretty much no-one, until operations for strabismus, or squint (ie a turn in the eye) were introduced around half a century later. Suddenly the minute anatomy of the outer eyeball became extremely important. Although other anatomists have since described, often in more detail, this fine fibro-elastic structure, it was Tenon who gave the first adequate description of it, and it has ever since been referred to as *Tenon's capsule*. The bulbar conjunctiva is separated from Tenon's capsule by the subconjunctival space (where blood gathers in a subconjunctival haemorrhage) except near the limbus, where the two tissues fuse. Thus Tenon's capsule is a sort of sheath for the eyeball that allows free movement of it without causing friction with the mainly loosely attached conjunctiva, and other structures.

Beneath Tenon's capsule is *Tenon's space*, containing an extremely fine meshwork of tissue fibres, which can be easily filled with fluid. Since all nerves supplying the eyeball must pass through this space to reach the eyeball, it is a relatively simple procedure to anaesthetise the eye for surgery by injecting the anaesthetic in this location. Of course, if only the front surface of the eye is to be operated upon, anaesthetic eyedrops may be sufficient.

The conjunctiva, then, may only be a lining of the inside surface of the eyelids, and a transparent lining covering the white of the eye but, if nothing else, think of it as the safety-net that stops contact lenses or other foreign bodies from disappearing 'round the back of the eye'.

CHAPTER THREE

THE CORNEA

'The eyes that shone, now dimmed and gone...' Thomas Moore.

Look at your partner's eyes again, or those of an understanding stranger such as you enlisted at the start of the last chapter. What do you see? The front of the eye appears to be white, with a circular coloured portion in the centre (the iris), which has a small, circular, black area (the pupil) in the middle of it.

Wrong!

Look again at the eye closely, this time from the side. You will now see that the iris is not at the front of the eye, it is inside it; a flat surface with a hole in the middle, like a Polo mint. In front of the iris is a transparent dome-shaped structure, of which the outline can just be seen, which actually is the front surface of the eye - the cornea.

The cornea forms one-sixth of the outer wall of the eyeball, the other five-sixths being the white of the eye, or sclera. The shape of the eye is maintained by the internal pressure of the fluid which fills that space between the cornea and iris (and some of the space just behind the iris).

Neither the cornea or sclera are quite spherical: the diameter of the sclera ranges between 23.5-24.2mm depending on which way you measure it, and the corneal diameter is likewise 10.5-11.6mm with an average radius of curvature (as viewed from the side) of 7.7mm.

The outer coating of the eye needs to be tough in order to protect its contents. The main constituent, collagen, is largely responsible for this toughness. The sclera has bands of collagen 10-16μm thick and 100-140μm in width which branch and interconnect in a complex way, with little discernible pattern. Individual collagen fibres within the bands vary between 0.03-0.3μm in diameter, with varying spatial separation. The collagen supports a matrix that consists mainly of a substance called chondroitin sulphate B, which is from a class of organic compounds called mucopolysaccharides (a mixture of complex sugars and proteins). Thus we have a tough, opaque (white) sclera.

All well and good. But the cornea is made of virtually the same material as the sclera. Yes, it is tough; but it is also transparent. How come?

A large part of the cornea's ability to maintain its transparency (which will be explained presently) arises from an extremely subtle difference in composition compared with the sclera: instead of chondroitin sulphate B as in the scleral matrix, the cornea has chondroitin sulphate A. These molecules have exactly the same chemical composition - they differ only in that two small units, totalling five atoms, switch positions. So, on the location of one carbon, two oxygen and two hydrogen atoms in a 55-atom molecule does the continued ability of light to enter the eye depend.

But what makes the cornea transparent in the first place? The answer is structural. Firstly, the cornea has no blood vessels to get in the way - although this poses its own problems, of which more later. Ultimately, transparency is achieved by the presence of a beautifully ordered, precisely arranged, collagen network. Remember that the scleral collagen is laid down in a more or less random mesh. Corneal collagen fibres vary in diameter from $0.024\mu m$-$0.04\mu m$ anteriorly to posteriorly but, crucially, they are finer than most scleral fibres and more regular in diameter within each band. The fibres are spaced with stunning uniformity at $0.03\mu m$ intervals, creating a lattice arrangement within each collagen band.

Why does this ordered arrangement matter? Consider a frosted window. The irregular patterns etched on the window cause light rays hitting the window to be scattered in all directions. This makes the window opaque because all we see is that scattered light bouncing back towards us. To make the window transparent we need to get rid of that scattered light. The situation with the sclera and cornea is somewhat analagous. The cornea makes use of the phenomenon of destructive interference to make invisible the scattered light. When two waves of light meet so that the peak of one is aligned with the trough of the other, destructive interference takes place; that is, they cancel each other out. The lattice arrangement of corneal collagen fibres, by being extremely regular, causes light to be scattered in a very particular way, one that results in lots of destructive interference.

Relatively large variations in refractive index (optical density) of neighbouring collagen fibres in the sclera reduce the destructive interference effect, resulting in increased light scatter, and opacity. The lattice arrangement in the cornea maintains very small refractive index variations, and then only over very short distances, so that destructive interference of scattered light is effective. The fluctuations in refractive index have to be limited to less than 0.2μm apart, which is half the wavelength of visible light: which is quite an achievement, if I may say so on behalf of the cornea.

Two main problems remain to be resolved:
1. How are oxygen and nutrients delivered to the cornea when it has no blood supply?
2. The concentration of different molecules in the cornea tends to attract water; but excess water causes swelling, disruption of corneal structure and, therefore, loss of transparency. So why is the cornea not constantly waterlogged and opaque?

In the next sections we will find out, but first we need to take an overview of the larger scale structure of the cornea.

Corneal Structure

The cornea has five layers, as follows:

1. Anterior epithelium - 50μm thick
2. Bowman's layer - 10μm thick
3. Stroma - 480μm thick
4. Descemet's membrane - 5μm thick
5. Posterior endothelium - 5μm thick

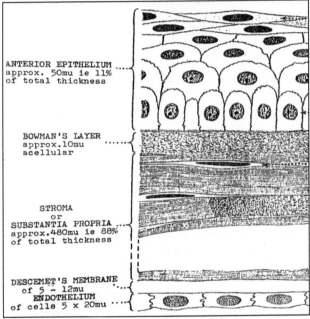

ANTERIOR EPITHELIUM
approx. 50mu ie 11%
of total thickness

BOWMAN'S LAYER
approx.10mu
acellular

STROMA
or
SUBSTANTIA PROPRIA
approx.480mu ie 88%
of total thickness

DESCEMET'S MEMBRANE
of 5 - 12mu
ENDOTHELIUM
of cells 5 x 20mu

Figure 3. Cellular structure of the cornea

Anterior epithelium

This is a type of epithelium which also occurs in other parts of the body subject to wear and tear by friction (in this case from blinking), but which is kept moist by a fluid (in this case tears). Comprising only 11 per cent of corneal thickness, there are five layers of cells, beneath which is a thin basement membrane of only $0.048\mu m$ thickness.

The bottom layer is continually producing new cells that migrate towards the surface, eventually peeling off to be carried away by the tears. In the surface layer, the cells have numerous tiny protruberances, called microvilli, which extend forward $0.5\mu m$ into the $7\mu m$-thick tear film.

The rapid turnover of epithelial cells promotes excellent healing ability: a surface scratch to the cornea will normally heal completely in 24 hours. A useful feature of the chemistry of the different cell layers enables an orange dye called fluorescein to be taken up by only the inner layers (where the surface layer has been scratched away); and it fluoresces a bright green colour under blue or ultraviolet light. This is one of the reasons for its common use in contact lens practice. The random fluorescein track produced by a particle rubbing around under a contact lens is actually quite pretty to look at (the owner of the cornea in question is not usually so impressed!)

Bowman's layer

This is a thin, cell-free layer, lying immediately beneath the epithelial basement membrane. It can be seen by electron microscopy to consist of fine collagen fibres of about 0.025μm, and it has enabled the name of Sir William Bowman (1816-92), the English anatomist and surgeon, also Professor of Physiology at King's College, to achieve immortality.

Stroma

The stroma comprises 88 per cent of corneal thickness. It is 71 per cent collagen by dry weight, arranged in bundles as described above. The matrix of the stroma, which occupies the spaces between collagen bundles, is made up of several types of molecules, including water, proteins, and our old friends, the mucopolysaccharides. One of the latter, keratan sulphate, is located at specific sites around the collagen fibres. These molecules have a high negative charge, and it is the strong repulsive force between them that keeps the collagen fibres in their precise position in the lattice.

Descemet's membrane

Descemet's membrane is, structurally, the basement membrane of the endothelium. It is unusually thick for such a membrane (5μm increasing to 10-12μm with age) and includes a grid of filaments whose composition is not easy to distinguish, even under an electron microscope.

Posterior endothelium

Here we meet another of the cornea's wonderful constructions. The endothelium is a single-cell layer comprising mainly hexagonal cells 5µm thick and 20µm across. The cell walls have many tiny projections so that the cells fit together like convoluted jigsaw pieces, the junctions being just leaky enough to allow the passage of selected molecules.

Cells, generally, are not replaced, so any gaps are filled by spreading and thinning of adjacent cells. So an older endothelium will have a greater variation in cell size and shape. Both of these effects can signal corneal distres and can be seen after long-term contact lens wear or corneal surgery. Endothelial cell density alters from around 4000 cells/mm^2 at birth, to 2000 cells/mm^2 at 80-90 years of age. The estimated minimum density for proper corneal function is 400-700 cells/mm^2, which is good news for centenarians, but a bit ominous for sesquicentenarians.

Oxygen In, Water Out

The structure of the cornea, as we have seen, comprises highly specialised layers of cells arranged in such a precise way as to make the tissue transparent. The two central problems of nutrition and maintenance of transparency remain.

Let us complicate matters first. There is a natural leakage of fluid into the cornea, across the endothelial barrier, from the aqueous fluid inside the eye. This provides most of the chemical nutrients required by the cornea. The stroma which, remember, is nearly nine-tenths of the corneal thickness, has a normal water content of 78 per cent and possesses a natural tendency to take up more, due to the water-attractive property of molecules in the matrix. So far, we have a cornea being flooded with water.

We can redress the balance a little. Ions (charged particles) of sodium pass across the epithelium from the tears to bind with the water-attracting molecules in the stroma, reducing their effect. There is also some evaporation of water from the corneal surface which occurs at the rate of $2.5\mu litres/cm^2/hour$; this can only happen when the eye is open, of course. The flooding has been stemmed, but our cornea is still waterlogged. What and where is the mechanism that keeps the cornea from being wet and swollen?

Studies in the 1950s showed that corneal water content, and therefore thickness and transparency, are temperature-dependent. A cornea removed from the eye and cooled would swell and become opaque, but these effects were reversed when the temperature was increased again. This showed that the water-removing mechanism was most likely a metabolic process, since metabolic activity generally increases when temperature is raised and decreases when it is lowered.

Where was all this metabolic activity taking place? By the early 1970s the evidence was pointing toward one particular structure. It had been found that on the insertion of an impermeable plastic sheet into the middle of a cornea, the anterior section would swell, but the posterior section did not. Removal of the endothelium of a cornea stored *in vitro* also resulted in gross corneal swelling. Thus the water-removing mechanism, or pump, was shown to be the single-cell-thick endothelium; a layer of cells less than one-hundredth the total thickness of the cornea.

Cell membranes have no mechanism for actively transporting water. Instead, the endothelial cells rely on a process well known to school biology students: osmosis. Where water can pass through a membrane, it will tend to move to the side which has the solution of greater concentration, until equilibrium has been reached. The endothelium was found to have a 'metabolic pump' which reduces the concentration of various ions in the cornea, by pumping them out into the aqueous fluid. Water molecules then dutifully follow along the outwardly increasing gradient of concentration.

In short, a precarious balance is kept between the inward movement of nutrients (which attracts water) and the outward movement of ions (which expels water).

Such a metabolically active tissue requires fuel - oxygen - that is supplied to other tissues via the blood. Remember, the cornea has no blood supply. For the answer to this, our second conundrum, we must move from the back to the front surface of the cornea. Again, in the 1950s, it was demonstrated that atmospheric oxygen dissolved in the tears is taken up by the epithelial cells. The microvillae (projections) of these cells, which extend into the tear film, aid the process. More recent studies have shown that, at night, when the eye is closed, a small amount of oxygen is supplied by the lining of the inside of the eyelids, which is richly served by blood vessels. Nevertheless, some corneal swelling occurs during sleep due to the reduced oxygen flow.

Oxygen depletion is really a double whammy for the cornea. At the epithelium, the metabolic process changes such that different waste products are formed than normal, which then diffuse into the cornea. Water inevitably follows. The endothelium has less fuel for its metabolic pump, also tending to create a net inflow of water. In extreme cases of oxygen deprivation (as occurs sometimes in contact lens wear), the distress signals are picked up by surrounding tissue, triggering the growth of tiny blood vessels into the cornea to provide an emergency oxygen supply. Of course, these vessels disrupt the delicate corneal structure, causing loss of transparency. And you're still tempted to over-wear your contact lenses?

Contact Lenses, Scalpels and Lasers

The cornea is not merely the window that allows light into the eyeball. Due to its curvature and being denser than air, it acts to bend and focus the light entering the eye. It is, in fact, the primary component of the eye's optical system. A corneal curvature a fraction of a millimetre too flat or too steep can result in an eye being long- or short-sighted.

49

Quite often, the curve of the cornea is not spherical like an orange; rather it is shaped like a lemon. The lemon-shaped cornea has two different curves - one steeper and one flatter - which results in two points of focus within the eye, most of the image being smeared out between these points. An eye with this type of cornea is said to have *astigmatism*. I have sometimes been informed by a patient that they have 'a stigma' - I think they mean astigmatism, but who am I to judge?

The idea of neutralising the power of the corneal surface by placing it in contact with water was exercising minds centuries ago. The earliest known writings on this subject are by Leonardo da Vinci (1452 - 1519). He referred to a transparent eye-shaped globe into which, on it being filled with water, the observer would immerse his face. Certainly, the optical power of his corneas would be neutralised, but hardly a practical appliance.

The next significant musings came from the philosopher and mathematician, René Descartes (1596 - 1650). His idea, a modification of da Vinci's, was to construct an elongated water-filled tube which, when placed in contact with the cornea, would create an enlarged image of an object on the retina. Again, having two long tubes of water strapped to the eyeballs hardly constitutes a convenient addition to one's lifestyle. However, there is a nice diagram of the appliance in Descartes' seventh *Discours* (1637).

It took a self-educated child genius to provide the stimulus to progression from optical theory to clinical application. The word polymath could be defined by Thomas Young's (1773 - 1829) career. He was familiar with twelve, and fluent in several, languages by the age of fourteen. He became Professor of Physiology at the Royal Institution carrying out research into, among other things, various aspects of vision. His investigations into the wave-like nature of light are still taught in schools today; his brilliant experiments on diffraction and interference of light are still the ones commonly used to demonstrate these properties. In 1814, his inspired lateral thinking and educated guesswork led to the deciphering of the symbols on the Rosetta Stone, the key to understanding ancient Egyptian hieroglyphs, which had remained a mystery since the discovery of the stone fifteen years previously.

Importantly for contact lens wearers, he had discovered astigmatism in his own eye in 1793, and his work of 1801 on this provided the basis for the investigations of the first of the Lucasian Professors of Mathematics whom we shall meet, Sir George Airy (1801 - 92). Airy himself was no slouch. Entered for Cambridge by an uncle who recognised his potential, he published his first paper aged nineteen, soon after he had become a Fellow of Trinity College. He was later Plumian Professor of Astronomy at Cambridge and became Astronomer Royal in 1835 - a post he held until 1881. In the latter post he played a major role in establishing Greenwich Mean Time as the internationally accepted standard. Building on Young's writings, he came up with the first optical lens for the correction of astigmatism in 1827, for use with his own highly astigmatic eyes.

The invention of Airy's lens in turn led to an important speculation by Sir John Herschel (1792 - 1871) that appears merely as a footnote in his dissertation on *Light* (1845). Herschel, the son of the discoverer of the planet Uranus, continued his father's researches in astronomy, was master of the Royal Mint for five years, and translated Schiller and the *Iliad*. He is buried in Westminster Abbey. The comment that concerns us reads as follows:

'..... it is worthy of consideration, whether at least a temporary distinct vision could not be procured, by applying in contact with the surface of the eye some transparent animal jelly contained in a spherical capsule of glass; or whether an actual mould of the cornea might not be taken, and impressed on some transparent medium.....'

Although the earliest contact lenses, at the end of the 19th century, were made of blown or ground glass, and covered the whole of the visible portion of the eye, problems with these led to Herschel's latter suggestion being adopted. However, one lens idea based on Herschel's first solution was put forward in 1886 as a therapeutic lens for post-cataract patients: the idea, from a scientist called Galezowsky, was to apply to the cornea a gelatin disc impregnated with cocaine and mercury, thus providing corneal anaesthesia. Perhaps he had been using the ingredients himself when the idea came to him.

Even with the greater comfort afforded by a lens produced from an exact mould of the shape of the cornea, there was still a major problem of getting oxygen to the eye. How often are the best solutions the simplest? In the late 1940s, the Hungarian physician, Joseph Dallos, and others, developed lenses with a hole drilled through them. Overnight, wearing times shot up from 4-6 hours to virtually all day. It is a truism in contact lens science that each development and solution to a problem throws up its own, often unforseen, problems; and these 'fenestrated' lenses were no exception.

We are now in an era of small (8-10mm diameter), highly oxygen-permeable, computer-designed rigid lenses, and soft lenses (12-15mm diameter) that may be 70-80 per cent water in content or made of new materials such as silicon-hydrogels (which promotes oxygen permeability). We have daily-disposable soft lenses: lenses that are worn straight from a sterile, sealed pack, and thrown away after use. Yet we are always seeking after the ideal lens to deliver perfect vision, comfort and health to eyes of all prescriptions.

But why not reshape the cornea itself? The degree of myopia present is largely due to the curvature of the cornea; flatten the corneal curve, and myopia is reduced or even eliminated. The idea has been around for some time in the contact lens field, using a technique called orthokeratology, where a tight-fitting rigid lens would push the cornea into a flattened shape. Versions of this technique still have their adherents today.

The first surgical procedure for altering corneal curvature was developed in Russia in the late 1970s by Fyodorov, although the first suggestion for such a method dates back to 1894. The procedure, called Radial Keratotomy (RK), involved making radial incisions around the central area of the cornea in a pattern like spokes of a wheel. The healing process would see scars formed which resulted in a flatter corneal profile. Obviously, the success of the operation was largely dependent on the skill of the surgeon. However, surgeon preference and the relatively low cost of equipment ensured that RK remained the most popular refractive procedure worldwide for some time.

The invention, by Professor John Marshall, a British vision scientist, in the 1980s, of the high-energy, ultraviolet-wavelength Excimer laser for refractive surgery, pioneered techniques for actually removing small sections of the central cornea to achieve flattening. The accuracy of these lasers is such that the cell next to the edge of the area being destroyed will show no damage at all. This process of removing a portion of, and thereby flattening, a central 5-6mm area of cornea is called photorefractive keratectomy (PRK) and proved a better option than RK. As laser technology has continued to evolve, other techniques in their turn have superseded PRK, such as LASIK (laser-assisted in-situ keratomileusis) and LASEK (laser-assisted subepithelial keratomileusis). Both these procedures essentially involve lifting aside the epithelium in order to reshape the cornea at the stromal level, before replacing the epithelium. There is also now a way of measuring accurately the minute undulations of the corneal curvature that give rise to minor distortions to the image formed at the back of the eye. This 'wavefront' technology allows the laser to be programmed to smooth out these undulations as the corrective procedure is performed.

It had been suggested, as far back as the 1960s, that any disruption of Bowman's layer (the layer between the epithelium and stroma) would tend to impede corneal healing. A technique of keratomileusis was developed where a central, superficial, disc of cornea was removed, frozen, its back surface lathed to the appropriate shape and then sutured back into place. It was performed in a few centres, including Moorfields Eye Hospital.

It is as well to look back to the story of contact lens development, and the delicate balance of anatomical and physiological factors that make the cornea work, to see how each advance brings with it its own problems. So it has been also with RK and PRK, although LASIK and LASEK generally appear to give excellent outcomes; but no doubt the cornea is yet to yield up its last secrets.

CHAPTER FOUR

THE FLUIDS OF THE EYE

'Every tear from every eye, becomes a babe in Eternity.'
William Blake

The eye is, as is the body as a whole, composed mainly of water. Here, we are going to look at the three fluids of the eye, all of which are well over 90 per cent water. Amazingly, it is the small percentage of each of these fluids comprising their other ingredients, that are responsible for their many and varied functions.

Cry Me a River - The Tears

One tiny little teardrop, trickling down the cheek: what a story it could tell. We only think about tears when we cry, or when our eyes water through irritation - but what marvels those teardrops are.

The volume of tears in the eye is normally only 8-10µl and, hardly surprisingly (and as mentioned above), they are composed largely of water: around 98.2 per cent water, in fact. But crammed into the remaining 1.8 per cent or so are a whole host of chemicals. To name but a few, there are: sodium, potassium, chloride and bicarbonate ions;

glucose and amino acids; proteins (including lysozyme, albumins and globulins); cholesterol esters, phospholipids, fatty acids, mucoproteins and, last but not least, good old mucopolysaccharides.

These substances all contribute to the numerous properties of tears. But tears just wet the eyes, don't they? Hardly. Let's now give our tears due credit by listing some of the things that they do for our eyes. They:

1. Provide the primary source of oxygen for the cornea - as   discussed in Chapter Two
2. Act as a lubricant between the eyelids and the corneal surface.
3. Have at least three antibacterial agents present, giving protection to the eye from infection. These include lysozyme, first found in the tears by Sir Alexander Fleming, the discoverer of penicillin, in 1922.
4. Help to remove corneal cellular, and other, debris, and foreign bodies.
5. Have a role in healing central corneal wounds, by providing a pathway for white blood cells to the wound from neighbouring circulation (remember, the cornea is avascular).
6. Smooth out irregularities in the cornea, improving its optical quality.
7. Help regulate the water content of the cornea.
8. Are a light-refracting medium; the first surface light encounters, and is bent by, when it meets the eye.

To perform all of these functions, the tears need to be more than just a quantity of watery stuff washing over the eyes. They need to form a uniform, stable film covering the corneal surface. This film is replenished and redistributed by blinking, approximately every five seconds. If blinking is suspended, the tear film will normally break up in around 15-40 seconds. That the tear film is stable at all is somewhat of a mystery since, given what is known about its composition, it just shouldn't happen. Various theories attempt to explain this phenomenon but, as yet, none have gained complete acceptance.

In 1946 Wolff proposed a three-layer structure of the tear film and, with minor modifications, it still holds good. First, a superficial, or outer, oily layer only 0.1μm thick. This is produced by modified sebaceous glands in the eyelids, called meibomian glands. There are other, smaller, glands in the lids called the glands of Zeiss and Moll, which may also contribute a small amount to this layer. An infection in one of these latter glands results in the commonly encountered stye, whereas an obstruction of the opening of a meibomian gland is responsible for the larger eyelid cyst.

The oily layer slows the evaporation of tears and provides lubrication as the lids move over the cornea. It also helps to stabilise the tear film in the manner of pouring oil on troubled waters; although, as mentioned above, this is not the whole story.

Secondly, there is a middle, watery layer. At around 7μm thick, this layer comprises over 90 per cent of overall tear film thickness. Most of this watery element is secreted by the lacrimal gland, which is situated behind the outer part of the upper lid, above the eye in the eye socket. There are also small glands in the upper inner surface of the top eyelid, the glands of Krause and Wolfring, which make a small supplement to the lacrimal gland secretion. The watery secretions generally decrease with age, which can lead to dry eye syndrome.

Thirdly is the inner, mucous layer. There is recent electron microscopy evidence for a two-part structure to the mucous layer, even though it is only 0.02-0.05μm thick. The innermost component is bound to the corneal epithelial surface and is possibly produced by the epithelial cells themselves. An outer, loose, component is produced by special cells in the conjunctiva.

The main function of the mucous layer seems to be to reduce the surface tension of the tears, allowing them to spread out evenly across the corneal surface. Otherwise there would be patches wetted by tears interspersed with dry spots: imagine a sheet of glass with some drops of water on it; only when something like a blob of soap is added, will the water spread out over the glass.

Many factors can upset the complex balance among these three layers. Reduction in secretions of the oily or mucous layers for whatever reason will destabilise the tear film, resulting in dry spots on the cornea or uneven tear flow. Hence the apparently contradictory explanation of watery eyes as being, in some cases, a dry eye problem; the eyes have plenty of watery secretion, but the surface of the eye is not being properly wetted or lubricated. This is like a window in a rainstorm, with rivers of raindrops running down the window leaving other parts of it dry.

Fine, I hear you say, but why, when I cry, does my nose always run? Well, about a quarter of the tears are lost to evaporation, but the other three-quarters have to go somewhere. Generally, the tears flow from the upper, outer area, due to gravity and the action of the lids on blinking, to the lower nasal eyelid margin. There is a tiny hole on the edge of both of the lids here (you can just see the lower lid hole if you pull your eyelid down slightly and look in the mirror). The tears are squeezed into these holes by the force of the eyelid muscle, from where they pass along small canals into a chamber, the lacrimal sac, juat inside the nasal cavity. From here, a siphoning effect pushes the tears down into a channel, the nasolacrimal duct, along the inside of the nose.

When you cry, there is suddenly a greater volume of tears than the drainage route can cope with; and it overflows, over the edge of the eyelids, and out of the nasolacrimal duct. So next time you cry, blow your nose and say a prayer of thanks to your tears.

Under Pressure - The Aqueous Fluid

The aqueous fluid, or aqueous humour to give it its proper name, is perhaps not so interesting for what it is, as for what it does. Suffice to say that it is very watery, of course - hence the name, *aqueous*. It fills two spaces in the eye, the anterior and posterior chambers which, together, have a total capacity of about 0.5ml. The anterior chamber is the volume between the cornea and the iris; the posterior chamber is the space behind the iris - between it and the lens.

The functions, then, of the aqueous are twofold: nutrition and mechanical action. It provides nutrients to several structures in the eye, namely the cornea, iris, lens and vitreous; as well as carrying away waste products. The mechanical action is the creation of an internal pressure to maintain the shape of the eyeball (much as compressed air maintains the shape of an inflated balloon). There's nothing too remarkable about all of that, except that these two functions require the aqueous to have opposing properties. To provide an ongoing source of nourishment, the aqueous has to be constantly formed, flow past the various structures, then drain away, taking with it waste material. But to maintain pressure within the eye, there has to be a steady, and sufficient, volume of fluid in the eye at all times.

The eye's solution to this problem is to have a drainage route that creates some resistance to the outflow of aqueous, so that with its normal production rate of around

2μl/min, the fluid is kept at just the right pressure to balance the tension in the slightly elastic wall of the eyeball - and so the eye stays its correct shape.

Observers as far back as the early eighteenth century had noticed that when the iris was inflamed, it would sometimes stick to the front of the lens. A billowing forward of the iris would be seen as a result of a build-up of pressure behind it, the path of the aqueous through the pupil being blocked. From these observations it was established that the aqueous is formed by structures called ciliary processes, behind the iris, and flows forwards from the posterior to the anterior chamber via the pupil. The manner of aqueous production at the ciliary processes is notable for the presence of a so-called blood-aqueous barrier; where some blood components, such as protein, are selectively blocked from entering the aqueous. The exact mechanism of aqueous production, however, is still up for debate.

To find out where the aqueous goes after its tour of the anterior chamber, studies were carried out, notably in the 1920s, which involved injecting dyes into the chamber to see where they ended up. Most of it found its way into a series of veins separate to those that the iris blood supply drains into. Some particles got lodged in a corner of the anterior chamber known as the filtration angle. Think of the anterior chamber as a dome, where the cornea is the roof and the iris its base. At the edge of the base, where the cornea meets the iris (as well as merging into the sclera), is the filtration angle.

The first structure that the fluid meets here is a meshwork, a loose arrangement of collagen bundles riddled with spaces. Let's follow the trail through the alien (and alien-sounding) landscape. At first, the spaces, the spaces of Fontana, are quite large (25 - 75μm wide). They then narrow to 0 - 8μm wide, increasing resistance to fluid outflow in the process. The fluid is squeezed into the internal channels of Sondermann, which lead in turn to the canal of Schlemm. From the canal of Schlemm the fluid drains into the external channels of Maggiore and onwards into the venous system. The progressive narrowing of the channels provides the resistance required to limit the rate of outflow, which in turn maintains the pressure of the aqueous in the eye.

The cycle of aqueous fluid production, flow and drainage with resistance normally works very well. But there are factors that can upset the balance, of which the most important is blockage - whether gradual or sudden - of the drainage system. When resistance to outflow of fluid is too great, because of narrowing or blockage of the filtration angle, the internal or, intra-ocular, pressure (IOP) begins to rise and this can lead to the condition called glaucoma.

To appreciate how glaucoma damages the eye, we need to return to our analogy of the eye as a balloon kept inflated by the pressure of the air inside (in the eye's case the internal pressure is provided by the aqueous). The key point is that the eye has a hole at the back of it into which the optic nerve is plugged, and the head of the optic nerve is a weak spot in the wall of the eyeball. An excessive IOP is therefore focused in this area, damaging individual nerve fibres as they fan out from the optic nerve on to the retina. The fibres that are damaged first tend to be the ones serving the peripheral retina, so blank spots appear initially at the edge of the field of vision - and may go unnoticed. If left untreated, the blank spots gradually enlarge and join up until only a small area of central vision is left, a state often described as tunnel vision.

The situation is complicated by the fact that some eyes seem to be able to tolerate a higher than normal IOP without any damage (a situation referred to as ocular hypertension), whereas others show optic nerve damage in the presence of a 'normal' IOP (so-called 'normal' or 'low-tension' glaucoma). The above is a very simplified account of the mechanism of glaucoma; in fact, the exact mechanics of what happens is still a matter for debate and further research. It is known that there are certain risk factors for glaucoma such as: age (the risk increases over the age of forty due to silting-up of the drainage channels); race (eg Afro-Caribbeans have a higher incidence); some diseases (eg diabetes); and family history of glaucoma, especially in parents and siblings.

Diagnosis in the early stages can be quite tricky. It is usually made from the results of three tests. The first is the appearance of the optic nerve head. The optic nerve head can be seen directly by looking into the eye with a special torch, called an ophthalmoscope, which is used to examine the inside of the eye routinely during a normal eye test (the ophthalmoscope and other imaging systems will be discussed in more detail later). Gross glaucomatous changes are easily recognised, although early changes can be difficult to identify, even with experience. The second test is measurement of the IOP. A variety of methods can be used, all of which, in effect, work by pressing on the eye to determine the hardness of the eyeball, much as you do when you press a fruit to determine its ripeness (the harder the eyeball, the greater the IOP). The commonest version of this test, which most people over forty who have had an eye test will have experienced, is the so-called puff-of-air test. The technical term for IOP measurement, in case you wanted to know, is tonometry.

In a sense, tonometry goes back to at least 1622, with recorded discussions of how to use gentle pressure of fingers on the eyeball to obtain a rough guide as to the IOP. This method, as I can attest to, was still being demonstrated to optometry students at least into the 1980s. Instruments that could take a quantitative reading of the IOP were developed in the mid-1800s. These were known as impression or indentation tonometers, as they relied on measuring the amount of indentation in the cornea that would be made by a probe under a given weight (the less indentation, the higher the IOP). A version invented by a Norwegian ophthalmologist, Hjalmar Schiøtz, around

1905, became a standard method of measuring IOP for the next fifty years or so. It had its faults and, given that the patient had to be supine, have anaesthetic eyedrops instilled prior to measurement and that the instrument's probe had to be rigorously disinfected between uses, other methods of IOP measurement were sought.

An alternative technique of applanation, flattening (rather than indentation) of the cornea by a known weight was pioneered in 1867, but it was an instrument invented by a Swiss ophthalmologist, Goldmann, in 1954 that was to become the 'gold standard' of IOP measurement, and remains so to this day. The Goldmann tonometer uses a small plastic probe to measure the weight required to produce a known small amount of corneal flattening when brought into contact with the cornea. It is done with the patient seated upright with the chin on a rest and, in skilled hands can get a very accurate IOP measurement in a few seconds. It still requires the instillation of anaesthetic eyedrops, as well as a fluorescent dye; the dye fluoresces under violet light, so most subjects' recollection of being measured by Goldmann tonometry is of a blue-violet light coming towards the eye. It is the preferred method in hospital eye departments, and of many optometrists too.

Even then, measurement of IOP is complicated by the fact that every eye's anatomical structure is slightly different; in particular, variations in the thickness and elasticity of the cornea can cause the IOP reading to be inaccurate, given that calibration of tonometers is based on average eye dimensions. To avoid such errors, the corneal thickness is often measured along with the IOP using an instrument called a pachymeter.

As explained above, the level of IOP alone can be misleading. The test of whether any vision has been lost due to damage of the optic nerve is measurement of the field of vision, which will detect defects in the visual field whether or not the IOP is within the normal range. This is done by the patient staring straight ahead into a machine that flashes lights all around the vision, the responses to lights seen being recorded. But the latest diagnostic instrumentation, notably the optical coherence tomographer (OCT), which is steadily spreading from the hospital ophthalmology department to the optometrist's consulting room, can image and assess the health of individual bundles of nerve fibres at the optic nerve head, revealing micro-damage even before the visual field is affected.

It is instructive also to have a good look at the width of the filtration, or drainage, angle in order to gauge the likely outflow of aqueous and the likelihood of blockage there. A rough idea can be obtained by direct observation with a slit-lamp microscope, an instrument commonly used in optical practice. A technique called gonioscopy allows a detailed look at the structures of the drainage angle also. This is done by applying a special lens to the surface of the eye, within which is contained mirrors that can enable one to peer into those corners. Should the drainage angle be narrow, there is an increased danger that it could get easily blocked or become closed altogether. This results in another form of glaucoma, termed 'acute'. Here the IOP can rise rapidly to a very high level, causing redness of the eye and symptoms of blurred vision and intense pain. At least, given the obvious symptoms, the glaucoma is usually diagnosed quickly – except when, on presenting to hospital Accident and Emergency, the patient is mis-diagnosed with an acute abdominal problem because the severity of the pain has induced vomiting. The condition is usually cured by making a small hole in the peripheral iris either surgically (*iridectomy*) or by laser (*iridotomy*).

Treatment of chronic glaucoma is by drugs that reduce the rate of aqueous formation, or an operation to open out the drainage route. These treatments are not cures; they only manage the condition. This is because the retinal nerve fibres, once damaged, cannot be repaired. And the volume of this little-thought-of, clear, watery fluid constantly trickling into and out of the eye is just (approximately) 0.5ml. Take a moment to go into your kitchen and look at one of your measuring jugs. It may be calibrated down to, say, 10ml. Then you will see how little 0.5ml actually is.

Through A Glass Darkly - The Vitreous

We turn now to the third of our eye fluids. We have looked at tears which flow across the eye yet form a complex layered structure of fascinating composition. We have looked at aqueous fluid flowing through the chambers of the eye, busy transporting nutrients and maintaining the internal pressure. The vitreous, on the face of it, just sits there: a bag of jelly.

The vitreous is significant because it is the largest structure in the eye. It occupies the space between the lens and the retina and is, from front to back, around 16.5mm in length. Its volume is 4ml, which is three-fifths the volume of the eye, and it accounts for three-quarters of the eye's overall weight. And it actually does quite a lot while 'just sitting there'.

Its bulk provides mechanical support for the eye and, when we look closely enough, we see that there is a constant diffusion of substances into and out of the vitreous; thus it provides nutritional support also. It is thought that there may be secondary functions, whereby the vitreous acts as a store of emergency rations for the retina, and as a dump for certain waste products. The latter function is implicated as being partly responsible for maintenance of transparency of the lens; there is both clinical and experimental evidence to show that abnormalities of the vitreous are, in some cases at least, associated with opacification of the lens.

The structure of the vitreous is a consequence of the sequence of its embryonic development. It is formed in two main stages, namely primary and secondary growth. As the secondary vitreous grows, the primary vitreous becomes compressed into a cone which has its base facing frontwards, at the rear surface of the lens, and its apex at the optic nerve head. With time, there is increasing compression of primary vitreous together with degeneration of the hyaloid vessels (those vessels that feed the embryonic vitreous). The result is the canal of Cloquet, a space lined by primary vitreous, containing the fragmented remains of the hyaloid vessels. The canal persists throughout adult life. The adult vitreous is mostly secondary vitreous, and comprises a gel interspersed with small amounts of fluid, the liquid vitreous or vitreous humour.

The liquid vitreous is 99 per cent water, which is bound mostly to one of our old friends, a mucopolysaccharide. In this case it is hyaluronic acid, a chain molecule that increases in volume a thousand-fold when fully hydrated. It was first isolated in the vitreous in 1934 and was given its name from the Greek *hyalos*, meaning glass, plus the fact that it contains uronic acid. (Incidentally, *vitreous*, from the Latin, means glass-like, the vitreous body having a glassy appearance.) Fans of mucopolysaccharides will be interested to know that the vitreous contains the most concentrated source of the stuff in the body.

The vitreous also contains very fine fibres of collagen (0.001 - 0.025μm thick), which interact with the hyaluronic acid. In fact, the hyaluronic acid is probably responsible for keeping the vitreous optically clear, partly because of the collagen interaction, which keeps the collagen fibres well dispersed (therefore reducing light-scatter - see the discussion of corneal transparency); and partly through its ability to inhibit the production, and invasion, of various opaque cells.

It may seem that the structure of the vitreous has been described in detail. But there is a lot more to it than mentioned above! Obviously, it is hard to see the minutiae of internal structure because, after all, the vitreous is transparent. Remove it from the eye, and it is difficult to keep track of what way up the wobbly bag of gel is. Since the eighteenth century, theories have been put forward for the minute structure of the vitreous, and the scientists are still arguing.

You may have an image by now of this bag of gel rolling and slopping around inside the eyeball. Actually, it is stabilised by attachments at certain places: at the forward margin of the retina, at the rear surface of the lens and at the edge of the optic nerve head. Which leads us on to those common visual symptoms, 'flashes and floaters'.

The vitreous becomes more liquid with advancing age, and this effect can loosen the attachments to the point where the gel becomes detached from the retina. The tugging of an attachment is thought to produce an electrical signal at that part of the retina, which the brain interprets as a response to a light stimulus - and a flash of light is "seen". When detachment of the vitreous occurs, pigment cells may be released from the retina into the vitreous. These cast a shadow on the retina, and the brain is tricked into thinking that the shadow has been produced by a speck of something *outside* the eye - this is a floater.

Symptoms of light flashes and lots of floaters may, therefore, be an indication of a vitreous detachment which, in some cases, can lead to the formation of a retinal hole or tear. This in turn can result in a retinal detachment. Vitreous detachments are relatively common, especially in later life, due to the increased liquefaction of the vitreous gel. But, by way of reassurance, retinal tears and detachments are quite rare.

As we leave our watery tour of the eye's fluids, I will leave you with one more fascinating fact about the vitreous, which is of no use to you whatsoever. Apart from the long list of organic and inorganic molecules that have been found in the 1-2 per cent that is not water, the vitreous has been found to have a varied metallic content, including (in alphabetical order): aluminium, barium, copper, iron, lead, manganese, molybdenium, nickel, strontium and zinc.

CHAPTER FIVE

THE PUPIL

'Beauty itself doth of itself persuade the eyes of man without an orator.' William Shakespeare

Strictly speaking, this chapter is about nothing. It's about a hole, the gap in the middle of the coloured iris. It has no colour itself, being a hole, but it appears black because it is the entry portal to the dark interior of the back of the eye.

The pupil reacts to many stimuli, by either dilating or constricting. There is an old story about a new medical student intake having their first lecture. The professor asks which part of the male anatomy increases by up to ten times in size when sexually aroused. A female student, keen to create a good impression by answering the very first question, states that it's the ……. well, the part that *you* were thinking of just now. The professor smiles and says that the young lady is either naïve or very optimistic because, in fact, the answer is the pupil of the eye.

Conveying subtle emotional signals may be important in terms of human psychology, but there are several optical reasons for a varying pupil size. Firstly, and most obviously, the pupil regulates the amount of light entering the back of the eye, which enables vision to function throughout a wide range of brightness levels. The actual amount of light passing through the pupil varies as the square of its radius (from the formula for the area of a circle: πr^2), which is to say that a pupil diameter varying between, say, 2 - 8mm (i.e. radius of 1 - 4mm) alters light sensitivity by a factor of x16. Which is pretty impressive in terms of optical imaging instruments.

Pupil constriction increases depth of focus, an optical phenomenon that improves the clarity of an object. Optically, this is most useful when viewing near objects. Perhaps our pupils know this, because they automatically constrict when we focus up close. They also constrict by reflex as brightness increases - which is handy, since aberrations due to imperfections in the eye's optical system (of most importance in bright light) are thereby reduced.

All of this is achieved by the balance of actions between the two muscles in the iris: the sphincter and dilator.

Wired For Light

The sphincter and dilator muscles are among the few muscles of the body derived from nerve tissue, reflecting the eye's formation from embryonic brain tissue. The sphincter is a circular band of muscle near the pupil margin of the iris, so that its contraction pulls the iris towards the centre of the pupil, making the pupil smaller. The dilator muscle fibres are arranged radially around the iris, like spokes in a wheel, so contraction this time retracts the iris, widening the pupil.

Each muscle is controlled by one of the two branches of the Autonomic Nervous System (ANS), the system that subconsciously looks after the body's functions. The ANS is analogous to an in-car computer which constantly checks that all of the car's systems are running smoothly and sends signals to modify the current set-up where necessary, leaving us free to concentrate on driving the vehicle.

The sphincter muscle, which is the more dominant of the two, is wired into the so-called parasympathetic branch of the ANS. It is this nervous pathway that produces the classic trio of pupil reflexes: direct, consensual and near. The direct reflex is a pupil constriction in response to a light stimulus. The consensual reflex is a constriction when the *other* eye is stimulated by light. The near reflex, as mentioned above, is a response to the eyes turning inwards to look at a near object. But how does a stimulus to one eye produce a response in the opposite eye?

To find out, we need to look at the neural circuitry of the parasympathetic connection to the sphincter. We start with the eye receiving the stimulus. The light is registered at the retina, and nerve fibres carry the signal out of the eye via the optic nerve - half of these fibres crossing over to the opposite nerve pathway at a junction called the optic chiasma. Further along, the pupillary fibres branch off from the main bundle of neurones bound for the visual cortex, to reach a body in the midbrain called the pretectal nucleus. From here - and this is the crucial part - fibres pass to *both right and left* Edinger-Westphal nucleus (a body that serves as the root of the IIIrd cranial, or oculo-motor, nerve). It is this double input to each Edinger-Westphal nucleus that connects the reflex responses of the two pupils.

The route thus far is known as the *afferent* pathway, the part of the circuit that carries news of a stimulus from the eye to the brain. The return part of the loop is called the *efferent* pathway.

The signal from one eye, then, has reached both Edinger-Westphal nuclei. Instructions to both pupils are carried by neurones contained within each oculomotor nerve, along with fibres bound for other of the eye's muscles. They reach a junction box, just behind each eye, called the ciliary ganglion, where they synapse with the neurones that carry the message to the sphincter muscle. That is the detail; the parasympathetic reflex can be summarised as a four-neurone loop:

1. Retina → pretectal nucleus
2. Pretectal nucleus → *both* Edinger-Westphal nuclei
3. Edinger-Westphal nucleus → ciliary ganglion
4. Ciliary ganglion → sphincter muscle.

Hence, a stimulus from one eye results in instructions for pupil constriction being relayed to both eyes.

Control of the dilator muscle is by the sympathetic division of the ANS. Activation of the sympathetic pathway originates in the hypothalamus in the brain, and results from psychological changes rather than from physical stimulation of the eye by light. The sympathetic route can be considered as a three-neurone arc, as follows.

One: from the hypothalamus, the neurone travels down the brainstem to a switching-station called the ciliospinal centre of Budge, at chest-level in the spine.

Two: from here, the second neurone travels to the superior cervical ganglion, in the neck. On its course, it passes close to the subclavian artery and the apex of the lung.

Three: the third neurone ascends along the wall of the internal carotid artery to join the ophthalmic division of the Vth (trigeminal) cranial nerve to reach the eye.

It is not hard to imagine, given all that circuitry, that there are many opportunities for things to go wrong. Pupil defects arising from faults in the system are normally classified as parasympathetic or sympathetic anomalies. In the next section, we will look briefly at some of the more interesting ones.

When Wires Get Crossed

Defects in the parasympathetic pathway cause a decrease in function, or paralysis, of the sphincter; resulting in an abnormally large pupil, through its inability to constrict properly.

The simplest case of abnormally-functioning constriction is the *amaurotic* pupil in a blind eye, caused by damage to the optic nerve. A light stimulus to this eye is blocked near the start of the afferent ('up-line') pathway, so neither pupil constricts. But if the good eye is stimulated the blind eye will constrict with the good one, as the efferent ('down-line') path to the blind eye is unaffected.

Most parasympathetic pupil abnormalities come within the classification of Holmes-Adie, or Tonic, pupils. The affected pupil is larger, of course, and, in fact, both direct and consensual reactions tend to be very sluggish. Interestingly, tendon reflexes such as the knee-jerk tend to be reduced as well. There is rarely a serious underlying cause – although that cannot be entirely ruled out.

Douglas Argyll Robertson published papers in 1869 describing a syndrome in patients with central nervous system syphilis, where the pupils would typically react better to a near stimulus than a light stimulus. Generally a bilateral condition, the pupils would be small and often irregular rather than large. Until recently, the Argyll Robertson pupil was considered to be a definitive diagnostic sign for neurosyphilis but, these days, diagnosis is normally confirmed by blood serum tests.

Sympathetic pathway defects result in a small pupil due to paralysis of the dilator muscle, which leaves the sphincter to work unopposed. The Swiss ophthalmologist, J F Horner (1834 - 86), has had his name put to a syndrome which reflects these defects. He is somewhat fortunate to be immortalised in this way because, although he described patients with symptoms of sympathetic pathway lesions, the general picture had been noted many times before, as far back as 1727, by Petit.

Horner's syndrome describes the affected pupil as being small; with drooping of that eye's upper eyelid (due to paralysis of a lid muscle connected to the same pathway); and decreased sweating on that side of the face and neck. Knowledge of the sympathetic pathway and the site of the interruption is crucial to diagnosis of the cause of the Horner's pupil.

For instance, someone with a Horner's pupil is often recommended to have a chest X-ray. Why? Look at the three-neurone pathway again. The second neurone starts in the chest area and passes close to the apex of the lung. A tumour there would damage that neurone. So could a breast tumour; or a neck injury; or surgery.

Diagnostic tests using certain drops in the eye produce particular reactions which can help differentiate among lesions that have occurred before or after the cervical ganglion (where the second and third neurones in the sympathetic arc synapse). For a pre-ganglionic lesion one might suspect one of the causes mentioned above. Post-ganglionic lesions suggest some kind of head trauma.

In closing this section, let me pose a question that may already have occurred to you: if one pupil is larger than the other, how do we know which is the defective one? Well, in theory at least, the argument is like this. If the affected pupil is the large one, the difference in pupil size should be more marked in bright light, when the normal pupil would constrict. An abnormally small pupil should be more apparent in dim light because it can't dilate like the normal one. Just thought you'd like to know.

Beauty is in the Eye of the Beheld

Come with me if you will to sixteenth-century Venice. We shall be so bold as to enter the boudoir of a noblewoman, where we find her surrounded by maidservants busy readying her for the evening's revelries. One maid is fussing with her lady's dress, another with her hair and a third is about to instil drops of a special potion into her eyes. And what's this? The concoction is a known poison!

Her ladyship knows that these eyedrops, made from extract of deadly nightshade, will dilate her pupils thereby rendering her even more beautiful this evening. If ingested, however, these drops could kill her. It is thanks to our Venetian lady of fashion, and others like her, that the scientific name of the deadly nightshade is given as *Atropa belladonna*: *atropa* from the active ingredient, atropine; and *belladonna*, meaning 'beautiful lady'.

Many substances, whether instilled directly into the eye or taken systemically, are known to have an effect on the pupil. The pupil can therefore be a useful diagnostic tool for determining what drugs may be active in the body. Other drugs can be used to provoke a pupil reaction in order to reach a diagnosis for a suspected pupil abnormality.

These different drug actions come about as a result of the wiring up of the two iris muscles, as set out above. To recap, the sphincter is wired into the parasympathetic nervous system; and constricts the pupil when activated. The dilator is wired to the sympathetic system; and dilates the pupil when activated. The key point here is that the two systems rely on different chemicals to pass on the signals from neurone to neurone to muscle across the gaps, or synapses, between them. A particular drug may either mimic, or enhance, the effect of one of these chemicals; or it may block the chemical's action.

Let me illustrate this explanation using the example of our Venetian belladonna. There is actually a family of belladonna drugs, which occur naturally in such plants as deadly nightshade (as mentioned earlier), henbane and jimsonweed. These are related to the tomato, potato and aubergine and contain as their active ingredient drugs such as atropine and scopolamine.

Atropine works by competing with the parasympathetic message carrier, acetylcholine, at the sphincter muscle receptor sites. Since it binds to these sites more readily than acetylcholine, atropine blocks the passage of parasympathetic nerve impulses to the sphincter, leaving it paralysed - so the pupil dilates because the dilator muscle is unopposed.

A drug such as atropine can be classified simply as a mydriatic, because it causes mydriasis - the technical term for dilation of the pupil. It can be further classified as parasympatholytic, because it blocks parasympathetic nerve action. Or, it can be classified as an anticholinergic, because it specifically inhibits parasympathetic action by blocking the signal carrier, acetylcholine. Note that we have started with one pupil, looked at two muscles and moved on to four types of drug action (enhancement or inhibition of each muscle function).

In fact drugs can be more minutely classified by their exact mode and site of action, for instance: atropine and botulinum toxin (one of the most toxic substances known to man) are both anticholinergics, blocking the parasympathetic nervous system. Whereas atropine blocks the action of acetylcholine across the nerve-muscle receptor synapse, botulinum acts further up the neuronal circuit, at nerve-nerve synapses. Clonidine, a drug used systemically to lower blood pressure, causes pupil dilation at yet another site, this time by indirectly inhibiting the Edinger-Westphal nucleus; which, if you recall, is one of the relay stations on the parasympathetic nerve loop.

Extracts from the belladonna plants were once the stock-in-trade of professional poisoners. A dubious use was once found for a drug with the opposite action to these. Physostigmine mimics the effect of acetylcholine by blocking the enzyme that breaks down acetylcholine after it has passed on a signal. The signals are thus prolonged until there is no more room for acetylcholine to pass across the synapse, after which the 'cholinergic' physostigmine loses its effectiveness.

Now follow me now to the Calabar coast of West Africa (in modern-day Nigeria). Certain tribes there made use of that cholinergic mode of action in conducting a type of trial by ordeal. They extracted a poison from the bean, known locally as the esere nut, of the plant *Physostigma venenosum*, which contains physostigmine. The accused would be expected to drink a potion containing the extract. If guilty, he would sip gingerly from the cup, expecting that the end was nigh. Taking it slowly, thus, he would end up ingesting a fatal dose of the poison. The wrongly accused man, sure of the immunity conferred by his innocence, would boldly gulp the potion down in one go, causing his stomach to vomit it back up.

Although out of favour as an instrument of justice now, the introduction of physostigmine into ophthalmology as a pupil constrictor was pioneered by Argyll Robertson, he of the eponymous syphilitic pupil syndrome.

A final thought: what have cocaine, LSD and caffeine got in common? They are all sympathomimetic drugs; that is, they enhance the sympathetic nerve signal to the dilator muscle, causing pupil dilation. So next time someone is looking at you and you see that their pupils are dilated, think: do they fancy me, have they just had a cup of coffee, or are they on LSD?

CHAPTER SIX

THE LENS

'The young men's vision, and the old men's dream!' John Dryden

Let me be blunt, now that we are reasonably well acquainted: you are not the person you once were. From the moment that you were born new cells have been growing, replacing old and dying ones. Eventually all the tissues of the body stop replacing the dying cells. Except one - the lens of the eye.

The eye's lens never stops growing. It increases in size and weight throughout life because the old cells are not discarded. The rate of growth is such that the thickness of the lens increases by 0.02mm per year. Whereas the central lens thickness of a newborn baby is around 3.5mm, by the age of ninety this will have increased to about 5.5mm. At birth the lens is avascular and without a nerve supply. As the lens grows, the older cells migrate towards the centre and become compressed.

Sir David Brewster (1781 - 1868), the Scottish physicist, was one of the prime movers in the setting up of the British Association for the Advancement of Science. He made important discoveries about the polarisation of light and, in 1816, he made generations of children happy by inventing the kaleidoscope. In the same year he published a paper in the *Philosophical Transactions of the Royal Society of London* on the structure of the human lens. It is rather sobering to consider that, despite the basic structure of the lens having been described so long ago, there is yet fierce debate over the fine structural details.

The basic details, then, are that the lens comprises a dense nucleus made up of newer, elongated cells, or fibres. This is the lens cortex. Then there is an outer, single, layer of epithelium. The whole is contained in a capsule, anatomically a basement membrane, the thickest such membrane in the body, varying between 6 - 25µm in thickness. So the nuclear cells are among the oldest in the body, yet are still more or less intact.

The material content of the lens is about two-thirds water to one-third protein. The water content is quite low compared with other body tissues, whereas the protein content is high - nearly double that of other tissues. This high level of protein in the lens presents a problem: whilst it increases the refractive index (light-bending property) of the lens, which is obviously beneficial, it should also tend to reduce its transparency. Of course, a high degree of the former is not much good without a good measure of the latter.

We are led back to the structure of the cornea and vitreous gel for the probable solution to this paradox. Transparency of the lens is thought to be achieved as a result of the very regular arrangement of the lens fibres, the effect of which is to minimise differences in refractive index between neighbouring sources of light scatter. These differences have to occur over distances of less than the wavelength of visible light in order for destructive interference of scattered light to be sufficient for transparency. Too much scattered light bouncing around in the lens renders it opaque to light trying to pass cleanly through. Despite the clever arrangement of fibres, however, the normal lens still scatters about 5 per cent of the light falling on it. This light is of a wavelength greater than $0.03\mu m$; light of smaller wavelengths is absorbed by the cornea.

The lens itself absorbs light between wavelengths of $0.03 - 0.04\mu m$, leaving only those wavelengths above $0.04\mu m$ to travel onwards to the retina. Light absorption induces chemical changes in the lens, including a gradual yellowing in colour; therefore, lens colouration is proportional to age. Yet again nature has done its homework because, although increased yellowing reduces transparency, it is also thought to act as an ultra-violet filter protecting the retina; and to help correct for chromatic aberration (unwanted colour effects due to spreading out of white light) inherent in the eye's optical system.

But what happens when too much colouration has occurred? Ultimately, the lens becomes opaque, blocking the passage of light to the back of the eye. The effect on vision is often described as like looking through a waterfall;

which is from where the name for this condition derives - cataract.

Cataract

It may seem strange to say, in light of the preceding paragraphs, that it is not known what actually causes cataract. Yes, we know about the natural yellowing of the lens with age, which results in cataract if it progresses far enough, but we don't really know what tips the balance - why, for instance, one person develops a clinically recognisable cataract while another person of the same age does not.

There are, at this present time, at least fifty anti-cataract drugs on the market worldwide (excluding the UK, where none have been licensed). To date, not one of them has shown proven effectiveness - the manufacturers would, no doubt, claim otherwise. According to World Health Organization (WHO) figures, cataract is the largest cause of blindness in the world, affecting somewhere between 30 - 45 million people. That's a big incentive for researchers and drug companies.

So what *do* we know? Risk factor number one is age, and the resultant exposure to many other contributing factors throughout life. We know that ascorbic acid (vitamin C), an anti-oxidant, has been shown to be protective to the lens; and this and other anti-oxidants such as vitamin E and beta-carotene may slow the progression of cataract. But it has also been seen that ascorbic acid can itself cause certain types of cataract. Equally confusingly, increased calcium levels have been documented in cortical cataract, but studies have shown that lack of calcium can cause cataract.

The effect of ionising radiation, such as X-rays, on the lens was established as far back as the 1950s and is a factor in cataract formation - but again, the exact mechanism of action is uncertain. There is evidence that microwave radiation can cause cataract in animals; the evidence for humans is more equivocal, but the potential for harm is there.

We are on firmer ground when we turn to risk factors such as diabetes - the link is well established - and drugs such as corticosteroids, phenothiazines and quinine which can produce characteristic types of cataract specific to each. Cataract certainly can be a consequence of other eye disease or trauma and can be present at birth (congenital) as a result, for instance, of the mother contracting German measles (rubella) during pregnancy.

There are many cataract classification schemes in use. It is an illustrative exercise to list cataracts by cause, as a summary of this section. It soon becomes clear from the number of causes (including some not mentioned above) how the WHO statistics arise:

1. Senile; i.e. age-related
2. Traumatic; i.e. resulting from injury
3. Metabolic; e.g. diabetes, hypocalcaemia
4. Toxic; corticosteroids, quinine, etc.

5.   Complicated; i.e. secondary to other eye disease
6.   Maternal infection; eg rubella
7.   Maternal drug ingestion, eg thalidomide, cortico-steroid
8.   Congenital, from other causes
9.   Systemic syndromes; eg Down's
10. Heredity; about one third of congenital cataracts are hereditary.

But it's not all doom and gloom. Fortunately, we can do quite a lot to remove the suffering caused by cataract - by removing the affected lens. Cataract operations of sorts were performed even by the ancient Egyptians. They did not remove the lens from the eye, rather they used methods to forcibly dislodge the lens from its proper position so that the cataract was removed from the line of sight. These techniques of 'couching' continued, with variations, through medieval times. Incidentally, the circa-fifth century Byzantine physician, Aetius, had a novel cure for cataract. He placed a whole, living, adder into a pot with fennel juice and frankincense; the pot was smeared on the outside with mud and burnt until the contents were ashes. These were grated and used as cataract medicine. It never gained much popularity (with humans or adders).

Until recently, standard cataract operations required a relatively large incision to be made at the edge of the cornea in order to create enough room to get to the lens, and for it to be removed through this space. The closing stitching of the wound tended to pull the cornea into a distorted shape, resulting in a spectacle prescription with large amounts of astigmatism. Moreover, as stitches became loose or were removed, the amount and direction of astigmatism would change. Remember also that removing the lens of the eye decreases the eye's focusing power by an appreciable amount - this also had to be corrected for in the post-operative spectacles, resulting in thick, bulbous lenses. Quite often, after one eye had been operated on, the patient would be left with completely incompatible right and left eye spectacle prescriptions (imagine looking through binoculars that have had one side reversed, so that it greatly diminishes the size of the object, while the other eye receives a magnified image).

An attempt was made some years ago to resolve these problems by replacing the cataractous lens with an artificial lens, or intra-ocular lens implant (IOL) at the time of the operation. The first IOL was implanted by Harold Ridley in 1949. Ridley, born in 1906, and whose mother was a friend of Florence Nightingale, became one of the most senior surgeons in the Services when he joined the Royal Army Medical Corps at the start of World War II.

After the Battle of Britain, many fighter pilots needed operations to remove splinters of shattered cockpit canopies from the eyes. Ridley noticed that these pieces of perspex never caused infections before removal, and this gave him the spur for an idea that he had had for some time: for implants as a way of solving the problems mentioned above. Most established surgeons were horrified at the idea of implanting something in the eye when the conventional wisdom favoured the removal of foreign bodies as a priority, to prevent possible infection. Unfortunately, because of the frequent complications which occurred with early IOLs, these were abandoned by all but a few surgeons in the 1970s.

Another solution presented itself at around this time, which was the use of contact lenses; or a single contact lens where only one eye had been operated on. A contact lens has the optical advantage that it can pack all of the required strength into a thin disc of material which sits on the eye, without the accompanying distortion and unwanted magnification that a spectacle lens of the same power would produce. The disadvantage is that most of the people in need of such a lens tend to be relatively old, making handling of the contact lens a real problem in many cases. The advent of extended wear lenses - lenses that could be worn continuously for weeks or months - seemed to overcome those difficulties; until, that is, the large number of corneal problems associated with such lenses became apparent. Although contact lenses can still be very useful, notably for infants after surgery for congenital cataract, by the 1980s the time was ripe for implants to make a comeback with the advent of a new generation of IOL material.

The modern implant has a size and power matched to the individual. Before the operation takes place, ultrasound measurements of the internal dimensions and curvature of the eye are made, from which the strength of IOL required to focus an image on the retina can be calculated. So whatever a patient's spectacle prescription is beforehand, distance glasses can often be dispensed with afterwards. Reading glasses would still be needed because, without the natural lens, the eye cannot refocus on near objects. Even these may soon become unnecessary as multifocal IOLs have begun to come into use. It is estimated that IOLs have saved the sight of around 200 million cataract sufferers. Among these is Harold Ridley himself who, in recognition of his invention, was knighted in the Queen's 2000 New Year Honours List, a year before his death. He was also honoured by Royal Mail when his invention of the IOL was chosen as one of six major turning points in twentieth century British medicine for a 2010 postage stamp issue.

The typical cataract operation today, using a technique called small-incision phakoemulsification, introduces an ultrasound probe into the eye through a tiny hole. The high frequency sound waves shake the lens to pieces after which the resulting gel can be sucked out through the same hole. The IOL, designed so that it can be inserted into the eye in a folded state through this small gap, is then placed into position. The initial incision is so small that only a single stitch - or sometimes no stitch at all - is required to seal it up. The whole process takes around half an hour, usually under local anaesthetic, so that most patients can, these days, be treated as day-case patients at hospital.

It is interesting to contrast current procedures with the situation at the beginning of the last century. I will let Professor L. Webster Fox, in his *A Practical Treatise on Ophthalmology* published in 1910, explain:

'The day before the operation the patient is given a warm bath, saline purgatives, kept in bed, and his face washed with castile soap and water. Two hours before the operation the skin around the eye to be operated on is carefully washed with castile soap; following this by placing eye pads saturated with a 1-2,000 solution of corrosive sublimate over both eyes ....The eye to be operated on should be thoroughly anaesthetised by means of a 5-percent solution of cocaine instilled into the eye.

The author prescribes 1 to 2 grains of mercury with chalk three times daily for a week or ten days before an operation.'

And after the operation:

'Both eyelids should be closed and covered with a generous amount of sterilized petrolatum, after which the small gauze pads and the large pad are applied and held in place by adhesive straps. A perforated aluminium guard .... is then fastened upon the eye operated upon .... Rest in bed in a darkened room for three or four days is always advisable. The diet during the first twenty-four hours should consist of milk or hospital soft diet....... The dressings should be removed at the end of twenty-four hours; the operated eye ....and the fellow eye is likewise bathed....... Both eyes are again closed .... and eye pads are held in place by a shield and adhesive strips. .... At the end of three days the unaffected eye may be left without bandaging, and at the end of a week the bandage taken off the eye operated upon one hour, on the eighth day two to four hours, on the ninth day and afterwards the eye is left open all day, being guarded by the bandage only at night. After this period dark glasses should be worn.'

Three cheers for modern day case cataract surgery.

Close Up: The Ageing Lens

We have talked about the structure of the lens and what happens when it becomes faulty, but what is the lens actually for? Perhaps that seems completely obvious: the lens - well, it focuses things, right? Correct, but in a specific way. You may recall that most of the optical power of the eye is provided by the cornea. But this is with the eye in passive mode, looking at a distant object, the parallel rays of light from the object entering the eye to be focused on the retina. What happens, though, when the eye needs to *change* focus to look at a near object? Extra power is needed from somewhere, and this is supplied by the lens. The act of changing the eye's focus from a distant to a nearer object is called accommodation.

The theory of accommodation was largely developed by Hermann von Helmholtz (1821 - 94), one of the giants of nineteenth-century science. Descended on his mother's side from William Penn, the founder of Pennsylvania, he held the posts of professor of physiology at Köningsberg, Bonn and Heidelberg, as well as that of professor of physics at Berlin. Some idea of the breadth of his discoveries concerning just the eye can be gained from the fact that we will meet him again in each of the next two chapters, when we will look at his contributions to retinal imaging and colour vision theory.

The accommodation theory states that the lens capsule has sufficient elasticity to mould the lens in to a more strongly curved shape (which is optically more powerful) when necessary. This elastic tendency is held in check by the normal tension of fibres called the zonules of Zinn, or suspensory ligaments. These zonules are arranged radially from the ciliary body - which contains the circular ciliary muscle - at their outer end, to the lens capsule at their inner end. The picture is somewhat like a wheel where the ciliary muscle is the tyre, the zonules are spokes and the lens is the central hub. The mechanism of accommodation is that contraction of the ciliary muscle relaxes tension in the zonules, allowing the elastic capsule to make the lens bulge.

The stimulus for accommodation to occur is a blurred retinal image. An afferent signal having been sent via the optic nerve, instructions are posted to the ciliary muscle along parasympathetic nerve fibres in the oculomotor nerve originating in the Edinger-Westphal nucleus. Some of this output is sent to certain of the extraocular muscles to enable the eye to be turned inwards for looking at the near object. The linkage between accommodation and convergence of the eyes is crucial in a number of situations that can give rise to headaches or eyestrain when the system is stressed.

Perhaps the most important case is when the available facility, or amplitude, of accommodation is decreased, as happens naturally with age. With a lower amplitude of accommodation, a stronger signal has to be sent to the ciliary muscle in order to increase accommodative effort. Of course, this has the additional effect of increasing the signal to the external eye muscles, so that the eyes tend to converge more than they really need to. Result: headaches and eyestrain. Problems of this nature usually start to crop up at around the age of 45 – 50 but are delayed in short-sighted people and tend to occur earlier in the long-sighted.

One remedy is to move the object further away, so that less accommodative effort is required to focus on it and, indeed, it is not uncommon to see people of this age-group resorting to arm's-length reading. The other option is to get help! Reading glasses will do the job or, for those already wearing a distance correction, extra strength in the form of a bifocal or varifocal addition to their lenses is in order. An optometrist could make a pretty good stab at telling the age of a person by the strength of their reading lenses due to the way the amplitude of accommodation diminishes with age.

Fransiscus Cornelius Donders (1818 - 89) was the first to set this out in a table of age versus amplitude of accommodation. His book, *Accommodation and Refraction of the Eye*, published in 1864, was very influential in the development of visual science. As professor of physiology at Utrecht, he did much to classify the different types of refractive (i.e. focusing) anomalies of the eye and laid the foundations of modern methods of sight testing.

The condition of age-related inability to focus on near objects is termed *presbyopia*, meaning 'old eye'. It is thought that it is brought about by a gradual loss of elasticity of the lens capsule which renders it less able to mould the lens to a bulged shape. This is not helped by the lens beginning to show increased rigidity with time. Either way, the ciliary muscle has to work harder to achieve a change of lens shape at a stage when it, too, may be losing some of its tone. As with so much to do with the eye, the complete picture is very much more complicated and has not yet been entirely elucidated.

Incidentally, it is worthy of note that those who have had refractive surgery to correct their distance vision and have been happy to throw away their spectacles or contact lenses, will still be affected by the age-related effects of presbyopia. Spectacles will once again be the order of the day, if only for near vision.

A final topic for thought: there is another way in which accommodation can affect the development of vision, or so it is claimed by some vision scientists. Over the years there has accumulated much anecdotal and experimental evidence to suggest a link between sustained near vision work (and, therefore, accommodation) and the onset and progression of short-sightedness (myopia). The question largely revolves around the system of nervous input to the accommodative apparatus, and its effect on feedback mechanisms which may exist to direct the eye's growth - a major factor in increasing myopia is an excessive elongation of the eyeball. It is no trivial academic matter, when one considers the proliferation of near vision tasks dictated by the ubiquity of visual display screens and mobile devices in modern-day life. Already the management and treatment of myopia comprises around one third of an optometrist's average workload.

Whilst the available evidence is in favour of a link between excessive near work and increasing myopia, there is less certainty, at present, of a causative action of the former towards the latter. Long-term studies hope to garner more information on the development of children's vision; other approaches are looking at the minutiae of the nervous inputs to the ciliary muscle. It may turn out that there are inhibitory nervous pathways which have a role in slowing the elongation of the eye by altering the feedback content to growth stimulation. If this is so, it may open the way to a pharmacological therapy for the retardation of myopia - a drug to stop short-sightedness. Some recent research has also linked inhibition of myopia development with the amount of time a child spends outdoors: exposure to natural daylight and less time spent focusing at short distances may be factors.

CHAPTER SEVEN

THE RETINA

'... for vision is nothing but the encounter of the eye with the powder of matter that strikes it.' Umberto Eco

It is at most half a millimetre thick, and lines the inside of the back of the eye. And yet here is the real business-end of the eye: the retina. The cornea; the iris, with its variable pupil; the lens, with its ciliary muscle and its zonules; and the various fluids of the eye, all exist ultimately for one purpose: to focus rays of light as efficiently as possible on to the retina. It is here, within the retina, that light stimuli are transformed into electrical signals that are then conducted by nerves to the relevant part of the cerebral cortex.

Indeed it is difficult to discuss the retina without speaking about the rest of the visual pathway. As illustrated in Chapter One, the retina is derived from the forebrain embryonically, the complexity of the retina and visual pathway being greater than any other bodily system apart from the brain itself. The retinal receptor cells that detect light stimuli are the rods and cones, so called because of their approximate shapes. Nerve fibres take the signals

103

which these cells transduce into electrical form, via the optic nerve and optic tract, to the visual cortex located in the occipital (rear) lobe of the brain.

A critical feature of the pathway is the crossing-over, or hemi-decussation, of half of the fibres from each eye to the opposite tract, at a site called the optic chiasma. It is fibres from the nasal half of both retinas that cross, so that the right cortex receives all the information from the right half of each retina, and vice versa. Something is wrong here, surely. Doesn't each hemisphere of the brain process sensory input from the opposite side of the body? Well, the eye's optical system forms an inverted image on the retina; so the right half of the retina receives information from the left side of the field of vision, and the left half information from the right field. And the general pattern of sensory representation in the brain is maintained.

I look inside thousands of eyes every year, and what I see I still marvel at despite the familiarity of the scene. Looking into an eye, assuming it is a reasonably healthy one, what one sees is the retina - because all the structures in front of it should be transparent. And it is beautiful! The retina itself is a deep orange colour due to its blood supply. It is a reflection of the retina in the pupil that causes the red-eye effect in a flash-photograph.

A major feature as we move around the retina is a light-pinkish oval area. This is a cross-section of the optic nerve where it enters the eye, and is known as the optic disc. The retinal artery enters the body of the optic nerve just behind the eye. Our view shows it branching out from the centre of the optic disc across the retina. The darker red retinal vein and its tributaries trace the reverse path. These retinal vessels will be discussed further in the next chapter.

The Macula: Centre of Attention

There is one small area of the retina, of about 1.5mm diameter, about 4mm away from the disc, which is not covered by retinal vessels. It is a shallow depression in the retina, near the centre of a yellowish pigmented area called the *macula lutea*, the yellow spot. (When viewed in a living eye the yellowness is not readily apparent, but the presence of the yellow xanthophyll pigment that gives the macula its colour can be more obvious in a dissected eye.) As I shine my light towards it, I see a small bright reflection. Within the macula can be delineated an even smaller area, called the *fovea centralis* – commonly referred to as just the 'fovea'. Here there are only cones, the receptor cells mainly responsible for detection of colour and detail (the rods specialise in detecting movement and faint light and predominate in the retinal periphery). The cones are tightly packed here. There are approximately 100,000 – 115,000 cones in the fovea; the more cones one has concentrated at the fovea, the sharper one's visual acuity is likely to be, all other things being equal. An eagle, for instance, has a very high concentration of cones in its retina, whereas an owl has a predominantly rod retina.

No wonder that so much time and energy is expended on remedies for macular degeneration. It can be such a debilitating disease because, although it affects such a tiny portion of the retina, the macula is crucial to providing the detail of everyday vision. One does not go blind with this disease, because useful peripheral vision remains, but central vision is impaired or lost. Just imagine wearing spectacles with a big dirty smudge of grease right in the middle of each lens.

The most common form of macular degeneration is age-related (ARMD), and it is seen more often these days because the general population is living longer. Around 30 per cent of adults over the age of 75 will have some signs of ARMD, while seven per cent have more advanced signs. The World Health Organization ranks ARMD third after cataract and glaucoma as a global cause of blindness, and the primary cause in industrialised countries. It was estimated that by 2020 nearly two hundred million people worldwide would have ARMD-related visual impairment. Some risk factors, other than age, have been identified, such as gender (ARMD is more common in women), smoking, prolonged exposure to sunlight, and genetic predisposition.

There are two forms of ARMD, dry and wet. The dry form is more common, and results from the natural ageing of a layer of cells that lies behind the retina called the retinal pigment epithelium (RPE). The job of the RPE is to provide nutrients to the retina and remove waste products. As it thins and breaks down with increasing age, it may no longer perform these functions sufficiently well. Deposits of waste products build up in the retina to the point where the cones are damaged and vision is affected. In some cases, the macula's lack of nutrition provides a stimulus for the growth of new blood vessels in order to replace the deficit (although the exact mechanism is unclear). These vessels are very fragile and liable to leak or rupture. This is wet ARMD, which by nature is of more sudden onset with a more dramatic loss of central vision. Subsequent scarring of the macula only worsens the situation. Dry ARMD tends to progress slowly but it is quite possible for it to develop a wet phase.

So what can be done about ARMD? In the case of the dry form: not a lot at this time, apart from ameliorating the symptoms with magnifiers, large-print books and other visual aids. Some early trials of treatment by argon laser produced mixed results. A process of essentially filtering the blood, called rheopheresis, has also been tried but its safety and benefit is rather doubtful. Other long-term studies suggest that supplements of combinations antioxidants and minerals, including large doses of vitamins C and E and beta-carotene and zinc may at least slow the progression of ARMD.

Photodynamic therapy (PDT) was developed in the 1990s as a treatment for wet ARMD. A light-sensitive dye called verteporfin is injected via the arm. It has the property of binding to proteins in the abnormal macular vessels, which are then destroyed when light from a carefully-directed low-powered laser is absorbed by the dye. The treatment is suitable only for a specific class of ARMD and needs to be given at the earliest opportunity.

PDT has now been superseded by the current treatment of choice, which is aimed at arresting the progression of wet ARMD and, in some cases, can actually effect a slight improvement in vision, is anti-VEGF injections. VEGF stands for vascular endothelial growth factor, a chemical stimulus to the growth of new vessels. Anti-VEGF drugs, injected directly into the eye with a fine needle under local anaesthetic, aim to block that vessel growth stimulus. Again, patient selection is important as the treatment is not suitable for all wet ARMD. More radical solutions have been tried, such as macular translocation, an exceedingly complex operation whereby the retina is, in effect, rotated so that the macula can be relocated away from the scars caused by the wet ARMD. And there is also a procedure that involves replacing the lens of the eye with a system of telescopic artificial lenses. It is not a treatment for ARMD but aims to maximise the potential of the vision available in both forms of the disease. It may be that stem cell therapy, by injecting into the eye cells that can grow into new, viable, healthy retinal tissue, will prove a fruitful avenue of research.

What about prevention of ARMD? There's not much one can do about one's gender. But stopping smoking and the appropriate use of sunglasses can help. As mentioned earlier, there is also some evidence that certain chemicals can have a protective effect on the macula. Vitamins A, C, E and beta-carotene have been implicated, as have the mineral zinc. Some studies appear to show that chemicals called carotenoids can also protect the macula. Dark green leafy vegetables such as spinach and kale are rich in xeathanthin and lutein, which are xanthophylls. As we have seen, these are organic pigment molecules that are present in high concentrations in the macula, giving it its yellow appearance. Lutein is also found in tomatoes, but in higher concentration in the cooked vegetable (which is my excuse for smothering my food with ketchup).

The Better To See You With: Development Of The Ophthalmoscope

I have several people to thank for my being afforded such a fine visual tour of the inside of the eye. It is only fair that we pay homage to them. I say *we*, since it benefits all of us that our eyes can be examined in this way. One can't just shine any old light into the eye and expect to see the inside in all its illuminated glory.

Imagine, for a moment, a ping-pong ball as the eye, with a small hole made in it to represent the pupil. The only place any light shone into this hole can be reflected out is through the same hole. And to see this reflected light, one's head would have to be placed directly in front of the hole - blocking the path of the initial ingoing light.

Our friend Helmholtz had the clever idea of moving the light source to one side, to be reflected off the front surface of a plate of glass tilted so that the light would enter the eye. An observer could then stand facing the subject and, looking through the rear surface of the glass, view the reflected light from inside the subject's eye. This very neatly removed the problem of the observer obstructing the light source. Unfortunately, the image seen is rather poor with this arrangement, as much light is lost in unwanted reflections.

An improvement was introduced whereby a silvered mirror was used to reflect light from the source into the eye, with a small central clear aperture for the observer to look through. The first mirror for this type of viewing system was apparently made by Charles Babbage (1792 - 1871) in 1847. Better known for his calculating machines - the precursors of modern computers - and another of our Lucasian professors of mathematics at Cambridge, he constructed his device by scraping away the central portion of silvering from an ordinary glass mirror. It was Helmholtz, though, who constructed the first instrument that could be properly called an ophthalmoscope, as these instruments are still called, in 1851. He also realised the potential of it and set out the underlying optical principles of its use.

The first person actually to view the retina was William Cumming in 1846, a year before Babbage constructed his mirror. Cumming (1822 - 55), an ophthalmic surgeon at the London Hospital, used a basic light source and reflec-

110

tor. But a very sketchy view of the interior of an eye was obtained fully twenty-three years before Cumming's attempt. It was achieved by one of the true giants of vision science, a man whose breadth of research in this area has left a legacy of several visual phenomena bearing his name to this day.

He was Johannes Evangeliste Purkinje (1787 - 1869). Born in Bohemia, he was professor of physiology at Breslau and Prague. His view of the eye's interior was gained by the simple expedient of using his spectacles as the reflecting medium for his candle light source. His eponymous optical phenomena are described in his snappily-titled book of 1823, *Commentatio de Examine physiologico Organi Visus et Systematis cutanie*, the subject of experiment often being himself.

Thus far ophthalmoscopes were a huge improvement on nothing at all but getting close in to the eye for a really good view proved difficult when the light had to come from a relatively distant source. The development of small, low voltage, electric lamps encouraged the next big advance in ophthalmoscope design; that of including, in the body of the ophthalmoscope, its own illumination. The first electric ophthalmoscope was constructed in New York in 1884. Present-day ophthalmoscopes still have much the same basic optical and illumination systems, excepting the addition of a wider selection of lenses and filters. The advent of small halogen bulbs by the 1980s improved the il-

111

lumination still further; think of how bright halogen car headlamps are compared with those of a few years ago.

The form of examination performed by the instrument described above is known as *direct* ophthalmoscopy. Another form of examination is now commonly used, called *indirect* ophthalmoscopy. It uses a different optical arrangement to view the retina which, though resulting in less magnification than with a direct ophthalmoscope, gives a much wider field of view and often a stereoscopic one too, thus allowing contours of the retina to be seen. The system relies upon a strong hand-held lens placed in front of the eye to form the image, with the illumination and viewing lenses being provided by either a head-mounted unit or a special table-mounted microscope that is otherwise normally used to examine the front parts of the eye. The practitioner just has to get used to the fact that the image formed that they see with indirect ophthalmoscopy is upside-down and back-to-front.

There has been a veritable boom in retinal imaging systems in the last decade. Retinal photography is now commonplace, especially in hospitals, whilst digital image-capture systems can display a retina on a monitor; the image can then be manipulated, saved for reference, or sent electronically direct to a specialist for an opinion. The latest laser-scanning ophthalmoscopes can produce stunning retinal images in the most difficult circumstances. Once more I doff my hat to Helmholtz, Babbage, Purkinje and the rest.

One Photon, One Spark of Vision

I quite understand if your enthusiasm for the retina is still, well, a little muted. Why do I get so excited by looking at one? Apart from, in my opinion, its inherent beauty, it is a remarkable tissue for a number of reasons. Without going into its ultra-fine anatomy, I would like to explore with you in a little more depth the structure of this amazing wafer-thin bioelectrical machine. For that is what the retina is: within its half-millimetre thickness comprising ten well-defined structural layers, it converts electromagnetic radiation in the form of light, via chemical interactions, into electrical signals that are then collated and processed and sent down the optic nerve. Which is all the more incredible when one considers that the design of the whole thing would seem to be back-to-front.

Wouldn't it seem obvious that, if we were starting from scratch, we would place the light-sensitive receptors at the front of the retina so that the incoming light hits them directly without obstruction? Underneath we would place the stores of photo-sensitive chemicals, and beneath these would be all the wiring, the nerve fibres to carry and process the electrical signals created by the receptors above. Not only is the reverse true, but nature has seen fit to place a network of blood vessels on top of the retina, as if wishing purposely to place an extra obstruction in the way of the light path. I shall return to these apparent paradoxes later to see if we can't resolve them, but let's now

113

turn up the magnification on our microscope a little further in order to find the point at which pure light begins to become vision.

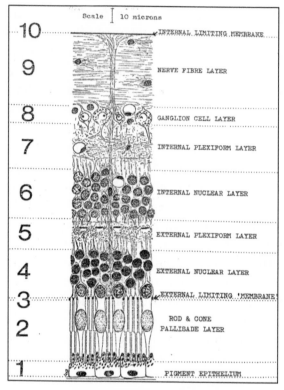

Figure 4. Diagram showing layers of the retina. Layer 10 is nearest the front of the eye; the retinal blood vessels lie on top.

114

It is the photoreceptors of the retina that perform this task, the well-known rods and cones - termed so, as mentioned previously, because of their shapes. They are arguably the most efficient and specialised receptors in the body. There are approximately 130 million rods and 7 million cones in the human retina. These are connected up to around 1 million nerve fibres; so it is clear that some data processing takes place within the retina, before the information even reaches the visual cortex of the brain.

In 1866 the anatomist Max Schultze described a correlation of rods with nocturnal vision and cones with diurnal (daytime) vision. Vertebrate eyes are built on a common plan but nocturnal animals, such as the bush baby, have pure rod retinas; while strongly diurnal species, such as lizards and squirrels, have pure cone retinas. Most animals' retinas, including Man's, are mixed.

The mixed retina has a central area dominated by cones, facilitating colour vision, high acuity and low sensitivity. In the human eye the cones are packed into this central area, the macula, at a density of 140,000 - 200,000 cones per mm^2. The peripheral retina has mostly rods; giving high sensitivity, low acuity and absence of colour. This makes sense in terms of the amount of light available during day- or night-time.

In the bright light of day-time the pupil is small, so as to moderate retinal illumination. And because the pupil is small, it is mainly the cone-rich central macula that is illuminated, resulting in sharp, colour vision. In the dark night-time, light is at a premium so the pupil dilates in order to gather the maximum available. Light falls on the peripheral retina, and the hugely sensitive rods respond. Altogether, the eye is able to function throughout a vast range of brightness.

The photoreceptors work by making use of special chemicals contained within them which react and change in a characteristic way when hit by a photon of light. And one photon is all it takes; research has shown that a single rod is so sensitive as to be able to be excited by a single photon of light, the smallest 'package' of light that can physically exist. A change in electrical charge on a molecule of the chemical in a photoreceptor cell takes place after it is activated by a photon and this is the moment, in a tiny fraction of a second, when light is transformed into an electrical signal: the signal which is eventually translated into vision once it has been decoded by the brain.

The photosensitive chemical, or pigment, in rods, called rhodopsin (visual purple), was discovered in 1877 by Franz Bell. It gives the retina a purplish hue when it is removed from the eye, as opposed to its orange colour when seen *in vivo*, due to its blood supply. The cones contain other pigments which we will discuss in the next chapter (where, incidentally, we will meet Helmholtz yet again). The whole chain of events from the impact of a photon on a pigment molecule, through the molecule's change, to its replenishment, has been minutely teased out by biochemists. My knowledge of biochemistry admittedly isn't too extensive, but it is a wonder to behold a chart of the chain of events as set out on paper.

The Back-to-front Retina

Such is the genesis of visual perception. Shall we now pull back to look at the larger picture of why the retina seems to have been designed back-to-front?

Let's first tackle the case of the retinal blood vessels. Here we have an immediate problem: with the vessels lying over the retina, shouldn't the vessels be constantly visible? In fact they are visible on some occasions, and Purkinje was the first to describe the resultant visible branching pattern obtained by shining a bright light into the eye from an oblique angle. You may have seen this yourself during an eye examination, created by an ophthalmoscope light being shone in the eye. The next time this happens you will be able to exclaim, 'Ah, there's Purkinje's tree!'

These shadows are only visible briefly and can only be maintained by constant movement of the light source; which leads us on to their explanation. The answer lies in the brain, and the manner in which the cells of the visual cortex are stimulated. The key is that these cells need a constantly *changing* signal to keep firing. This mechanism helps, among other things, to weed out redundant information thereby avoiding sensory overload. The shadow of the pattern of retinal vessels normally always falls on the same retinal receptors, resulting in an *unchanging* signal being received by their corresponding cortical cells. The cortical cells stop firing, and the shadows disappear.

It is possible to see this cortical adaptation by looking very still at a single star in the night sky with one eye. Eventually the star will seem to fade away but will return immediately on the slightest movement of the eye. The visual system actually has a built-in a mechanism of constant tiny eye movements in order to ensure regular re-stimulation of the cortical cells; otherwise we'd find that our normal visual image would have a tendency to keep fading (see Chapter Nine).

By way of a small digression, Purkinje was also the first to describe another phenomenon thought to be due to the structure of the retina. It is one of my favourite entoptic images (as images produced within optical structures are called) because it is rather beautiful and quite easy to envisage. One needs to look at a small, preferably red, light, in the dark. I find the LED standby light on a television or set-top box is very good for this, but a red car tail-light sometimes works. An effect should appear of bluish-purple arcs curving out from the top and bottom of the light. Small eye movements help prolong the image, which is thought to result from the radial pattern of nerve fibre bundles in the retina.

What a wonderful 'software solution Nature has provided to a vital 'hardware arrangement; for the overlying retinal vessels give the retina a double blood supply. They provide the upper neuronal layers of the retina with nourishment while the blood-rich underlying tissue, the cho-roid, supplies the photoreceptor layers.

Out in the Visual Field – Part One

The field of vision of the eye, meaning the extent in all directions the eye can see when looking straight ahead, is mapped onto the retina as described before. Everything in the visual field to the right of centre is mapped onto the left side of the retina, to be interpreted by the left visual cortex; and vice versa. But there is a great big black hole of blindness within this field, corresponding to the area at the back of the eye where the optic nerve enters. Here there are no retinal photoreceptors, so an image cannot be formed at this site.

We can find the blind spot by making a plot of the ex-tent of the visual field. This is done by moving a target or flashing a light at various points in front of the eye and mapping the places where the stimulus is seen. Each place corresponds to a specific point on the retina, so such a plot will show up the oval void in the visual field that matches up with the optic disc.

So why don't we see two blank blobs in our vision all the time? It is partly because of constant eye movements which move the blind spot around so that it doesn't persis-tently block out the same object. Also, the blind spot for each eye falls within the visual field of the other eye so, in effect, each eye sees what is hidden by the other eye's blind spot; the gaps are filled in. Another clever solution by Nature.

Let's now turn to another aspect of the relationship of vision with the retina. Picture a cross-section of an eye: the eye is sliced horizontally through the middle and we look down on the half that remains after the top is removed. We then draw a line through the centre of the cornea and lens, dividing our cross-section in half. This line, continued, intersects the retina, amazingly, not at the macula, the central and most sensitive part, corresponding to the centre of the visual field!

If we draw another line from the macula back out to the centre of the visual field we find that the angle between this, the visual axis, and the former line, the optical axis, is approximately 5 degrees. One would naturally expect the two lines to be one and the same; to be superimposed. But because the eye's optical and visual axes are misaligned, any point fixated upon is viewed obliquely to the optical system. It is almost as if one decides to use a telescope by looking into the eyepiece slightly from one side.

Has Nature gone mad? This discrepancy, not surprisingly, is responsible for introducing certain kinds of optical aberration into the visual image. Some is corrected for by the curvature of the cornea and lens, and the variability of pupil size. But some remains, in the form of the production of a slightly elongated, smeared out, focus as opposed to a perfect point focus.

It turns out that this is quite useful because it leaves some leeway if the length of the eye is not ideal. In other words, the eye will still be more or less in focus even if the eyeball is a touch too long or short for light to be brought to an exact focus on the retina. The tolerance is enough for a small adjustment in accommodation to be able to bring the image back into sharper definition; the eye does not suddenly have to be declared long- or short-sighted for minor errors in eye length.

How clever is that? The obvious way to design the eye (or any optical instrument) would be to reduce optical aberrations to a minimum and focus the image as sharply and accurately as possible. Nature has found that this is not necessarily the best solution for achieving a highly flexible visual system, so I apologise to her for questioning her sanity. My faith (and yours, I hope) in Nature is restored.

CHAPTER EIGHT

THE BLOOD VESSELS OF THE EYE

'My eyes make pictures, when they are shut.' Samuel Taylor Coleridge

Let me state at the outset one of the most remarkable and important facts about the eye (thanks to those pioneers mentioned in the previous chapter who invented ways of looking into the eye): it is the only place in the body where one can view directly arteries and veins.

Blood vessels can be seen, in a way, under the skin or even on the surface of the eye but, in both cases, they are covered by tissue. True, the conjunctiva that covers the vessels seen on the white of the eye (sclera) is transparent, but these vessels are only small capillaries. What can be seen at the back of the eye with an ophthalmoscope, through transparent media, are full-blown, pukka arteries and veins and, as such, they provide a direct commentary on the body's cardiovascular system and its state of health.

Many general health conditions affecting the heart and the circulatory apparatus of arteries, veins and small capillaries, can leave clues to their presence in the appearance of the retinal vessels. Some of the more common ones include hypertension (high blood pressure), arteriosclerosis (hardening of the arteries), raised cholesterol and diabetes. In all these cases observation of the retina may be the first sign of the disease in an otherwise asymptomatic patient. Good examples of this, though of rarer occurrence than those conditions just mentioned, are carotid artery and cardiac valve stenosis (narrowing), in which the ophthalmic signs may be the first indication of quite advanced arterial or heart disease.

All the above serves to emphasise why it is so important to have a regular eye examination. A two-minute perusal of the retinal vessels could reveal an otherwise-unsuspected threat of heart disease or stroke; not to mention brain lesions or lung tumours, neurological conditions and eye diseases that other parts of the eye examination can detect.

A closer look at the blood supply to the eye will help to show why it is such an important signpost to the body's health. The eye is supplied with (oxygenated) blood via the ophthalmic artery, which is a major branch of the internal carotid artery, itself a division of the common carotid artery which supplies the head and neck. The common carotid originates in the arch of the aorta (there are anatomical variations between right and left carotids), the largest artery in the body, arising from the left ventricle of the heart. So the ophthalmic artery is only three 'steps' from the largest artery in the body, and the central retinal ar-

'

tery, which is the main artery that can be seen in the eye, is a direct branch of that. Also, since the carotids supply both the eyes and brain, anything that affects the eyes' circulation potentially could affect the brain (and vice versa), another of the reasons that examination of the retinal vessels is so important.

The ophthalmic artery itself has many branches. These are usually classified by whether they supply parts of the eye, the *ocular group*, or its surrounding structures, the *orbital group*. The orbital group is of less interest to us here, suffice to say that these branches supply the lacrimal gland, eyelids, forehead, nose and other structures in and around the orbit. We will concentrate on the ocular group.

Purkinje's Tree

In the last chapter we met Purkinje's tree as a description of the shadow cast on the retina by the retinal vessels when a light is shone into the eye at an unusual, oblique, angle. Now we will take a look at the vessels themselves.

The central retinal artery enters the sheath of the optic nerve just behind the eyeball. As it enters the eye it sends branches to serve all four quadrants of the retina except the fovea and its immediate surrounds within the macula. The branches divide further into smaller and smaller vessels, the smallest being termed capillaries. The retinal arteries in fact only supply the inner layers of the retina, accounting for 20-30 per cent of the retina's total blood supply. The rest is provided by another part of the ocular circulatory system which is quite separate from the retinal supply but which also arises from the ocular group of ophthalmic artery branches, and which will be described shortly.

Two examples will serve to show how a basic examination of the retinal vessels can indicate the presence of cardiovascular disease: retinal artery embolism and retinal vein occlusion. A sudden painless loss of vision in one eye is usually experienced with central retinal artery blockage, or occlusion. The occlusion may be caused by an embolism, which could be a blood clot or a plaque of cholesterol. These emboli typically break away from the inner lining of a larger, diseased, blood vessel and travel through the blood stream until they reach an artery too narrow to pass through. The carotid artery is often the origin of such cholesterol plaques, so it is no surprise that they often reach the retinal arteries. If an embolism makes it further into the retinal circulation, blockage may occur at one of the smaller branches, causing just a sector of vision to be lost that may not be noticed by the sufferer, who remains oblivious to the condition until the occlusion is spotted by examination. The three major concerns are of permanent vision loss if the condition is not treated urgently, undiagnosed cardiovascular disease and danger of potential stroke caused by an embolism lodging in one of the cerebral arteries.

Sometimes an examiner may see a bright shiny yellow blob sitting in one of the smaller retinal arteries. It is likely to be asymptomatic and may not be causing a complete occlusion of the vessel, so the retina around it is unaffected. These rather beautiful Hollenhorst plaques, named after the American ophthalmologist who first realised their significance, are small cholesterol emboli that are usually pieces of larger plaques originating in the internal carotid, so their presence should prompt investigation of that important vessel.

Retinal vein occlusion is also often characterised by one eye's sudden painless loss of vision. The main causes are blood clot (thrombus) and high blood pressure (hypertension). Whereas thrombus causes a direct blockage of the vein, in hypertension a vein is compressed by a 'stiffened' artery crossing over it. There are many such artery-over-vein crossings of the retinal vessels; careful study of these for early signs of 'pinching' or 'nipping' of the veins is a regular part of the optometrist's routine examination of the retina. If it has ever been suggested to you after an eye examination to have your blood pressure checked, it is most likely to be as a result of seeing such signs, or perhaps a suspicious change in the normal ratio of artery/vein thickness or excessive 'wiggliness' of the vessels; or maybe all three.

Retinal vein occlusion is the second most common retinal vascular disorder after diabetic retinal disease and until recently there was no treatment for it. Argon laser treatment has been found to be of limited help, and new anti VEGF therapy licensed for this particular use is proving somewhat more successful. Otherwise, management consists of checking relevant general health factors, such as possible hypertension, and monitoring the eye for possible complications, such as glaucoma. Vision may improve somewhat over time, depending on how badly it is affected in the first place.

But mention should be made also of diabetic eye disease since, as stated above, it is the most common ocular vascular disease – and still a major cause of largely preventable blindness. The length of time diabetes has been present and poor control of the condition are the main risk factors for the onset of retinal disease. Diabetes causes changes to the blood vessel walls which can result in localised swellings, or microaneurysms, of the fine retinal vessels, seen as little spots of blood on the retina. This may cause malnourishment of parts of the retina, with associated leaking out of proteins from the vessels, yellowish patches called exudates. Prolonged deprivation of oxygen resulting from lack of blood flow to retinal areas stimulates the growth of new vessels to take up the slack; but these vessels tend to be very fragile and haemorrhage easily. Such haemorrhages ultimately can cause glaucoma and detached retina. The earlier diabetic retinopathy is diagnosed, the easier it is to manage, thus avoiding the more severe complications. This is why diabetics are allowed an annual NHS eye examination with an optometrist, as well as having an annual diabetic eye screening in which digital photographs are taken of the retina that can be graded and compared with previous years' images.

The beautiful array of retinal arteries and veins spreading out like branches of a tree from the optic disc, that can be viewed via an ophthalmoscope (or other imaging system), appears to vary infinitely among individuals while based on a fairly standard template. Indeed, it was suggested by researchers Simon and Goldstein as far back as 1935 that, because the course and distribution of the branches of the retinal vessels does vary so much, these retinal patterns may be so individualistic as to be useful in the identification of criminals. The doyen of twentieth century ophthalmologists, Sir Stewart Duke-Elder, GVCO, MA, LLD, PhD, DSc, MD, FRCS, FRCS(Edin), FACS, FRACS, FRCP, FRS, writing in his monumental work, *System of Ophthalmology*, in 1961 says, with little perception of future technological developments, 'Fundus [ie retinal] photography would appear to be a rather elaborate procedure as compared with the simple recording of finger-prints!' Note the dismissive exclamation mark at the end. In fact, digital fundus photography is now available in many 'high street' optical practices, let alone its everyday use in hospital eye departments. While the technology is still rather expensive and less portable than fingerprinting, it may yet find a place in the canon of identification techniques as has iris pattern recognition in some security applications.

Duke-Elder (1898 – 1978), it is worth pointing out, was one of the main authorities antagonistic to Harold Ridley's idea of implanting an artificial lens after cataract removal, that we looked at in Chapter Six. He may have been proved wrong ultimately in that argument, but his achievements in ophthalmology were significant. During his time studying at St Andrews University he gained a BSc with distinction in physiology and in the same year an MA with first class honours in natural science; and was awarded a gold medal for his MD thesis. By the age of twenty-seven he was honorary consulting surgeon at both St George's and Moorfields hospitals in London. In 1932 he operated on the Prime Minister, Ramsay MacDonald, a glaucoma sufferer and, in the same year, began work on a seven-volume book, *Text-Book of Ophthalmology*, which took twelve years to complete.

Duke-Elder soon decided that his *Text-Book* was in need of updating, so in 1958 he began work on the aforementioned *System of Ophthalmology* which, with collaborators, was to encompass every conceivable branch of the subject, running to fifteen volumes. It was finally completed in 1976 and is still widely referred to (including by me for this book). He also helped to create the Institute of Ophthalmology which opened in 1948 and, being closely associated with Moorfields, is now a world-renowned research facility. Another of his achievements was the formation of the faculty of ophthalmologists within the Royal College of Surgeons, serving as its first president. Overseas, he helped to open a new hospital of St John of Jerusalem in 1960. Yet he found time to be the longest holder of the post of Surgeon Oculist to the royal family, serving three monarchs in twenty-nine years.

It could be said fairly that he helped to shape modern ophthalmology in Britain, but the battle with Ridley is a salutary illustration that in science generally, deference to authority or consensus is - or, at least, should be - no match for the argument of actual experimental observations and the logical presentation of facts.

The Retina's Coat – the Choroid

Sandwiched between the retina and the outer coating of the eye, the sclera, lies a thin tissue, approximately 0.1mm thick, called the choroid. Its primary function is to provide a blood supply to the outer layers of the retina and the fovea and its immediate surrounds – remember it was mentioned above that the retinal vessels only supply the inner retinal layers and the macula not at all.

The choroid's blood vessels derive from the ciliary arteries which, like the retinal vessels are branches of the ophthalmic artery. There are long and short posterior ciliary arteries: the long posterior ciliary arteries pass forward to supply the iris and other ocular structures, including the anterior choroid, while the short posterior ciliary arteries are responsible for the majority of the choroidal blood supply. These arteries perform an intricate dance as they enter the sclera in a circular pattern around the optic nerve at the rear of the eyeball. They join up to form a circular structure surrounding the optic nerve, called the *cir-*

cle of Zinn. Like the exits of the M25 motorway, there are vessels that branch off regularly to reach the choroid, along with some direct short posterior ciliary branches from the ophthalmic artery that do not contribute to the circle of Zinn.

Within the choroid the arteries begin branching rapidly. The area nearest the sclera is composed of, firstly, largish vessels, sometimes referred to as *Haller's layer* after the eighteenth-century anatomist, Albrecht Haller who, incidentally, composed the world's first comprehensive work on human physiology. Next is a layer of small vessels, known as *Sattler's layer*, named after the early nineteenth-century ophthalmologist, Hubert Sattler, who is recognised for his definitive work on the histology of the choroid. From here the arteries move perpendicularly inwards and break up suddenly into star-shaped formations of capillaries that radiate out in all directions in a layer called the *choriocapillaris*. These capillaries are unusual in size; compared with those found in other organs, they are extremely wide, allowing several red blood cells to pass through side by side compared with the normal one-cell capillary width. The network of capillaries is also unusual in that it spreads out in a single plane rather than, to use a rough analogy, forming a sponge-like meshwork.

The choriocapillaris is intimately connected with a structure called *Bruch's membrane*, a fibrous, elastic tissue that forms the basement membrane of the retinal pigment epithelium, the outermost layer of the retina. It is through

Bruch's membrane that oxygen and other nutrients must pass from the choriocapillaris to the outer retina. The surface of the choriocapillaris facing Bruch's membrane is punctured by many tiny openings, each covered by a diaphragm, through which molecules may pass.

Wet age-related macular degeneration (ARMD), which we looked at in the previous chapter, can now be visualised from the other side, so to speak. It is characterised by an abnormal proliferation of the capillaries of the choriocapillaris, which sometimes break through Bruch's membrane at the macula. Leakage of blood or other fluids from these vessels will most likely cause detachment of the retina or its pigment epithelium, resulting in loss of central vision. Treatment of wet ARMD by injection aims to inhibit the growth factor that appears to be responsible for the abnormal vessel growth.

Originally the adjacent structures of the retinal pigment epithelium, Bruch's membrane and choriocapillaris, were known collectively as *tunica Ruyschiana* after the Dutch physician and botanist, Frederick Ruysch (1638 – 1731), who was professor of anatomy at Amsterdam. He invented a method of injecting vessels with a solution, later revealed to be a mixture of talc, white wax and cinnabar, that enabled him to describe the vascular system of the eye as well as much other human anatomy. He preserved his specimens in an embalming fluid comprised of alcohol (from wine or corn) with a dash of black pepper. He built up a huge collection of specimens which, in 1717, was sold to Tsar Peter the Great for 30,000 guilders. It was rumoured that only a few specimens reached St Petersburg due to sailors drinking the preserving spirits *en route*, but in fact the collection arrived in tact.

The oxygen and nutrients supplied to the retina by the choroid aid metabolism and healthy functioning of the outer retina. Of course, all the waste products produced by this metabolic activity, particularly of the retinal photoreceptors, has to be removed somehow. Thus there is a transport of material back across Bruch's membrane to be carried away by the choroidal venous system.

The Return Journey – the Venous System

Let us begin the return journey, the route taken by the now deoxygenated blood, at the point we have just reached – the choriocapillaris. Small veins, called venules, arise from the choriocapillaris, which merge into increasingly larger veins that pass to the outer choroidal layer. The larger veins in each quadrant of the choroid then converge to form a vortex, or vertical, vein. The four vortex veins arise at roughly the equator of the eye, that is, about half way from the back and the front. They travel a little way through canals in the sclera to emerge from the eyeball somewhat posterior to the equator at about ninety degrees away from each other.

The two superior vortex veins and the two inferior vortex veins empty into the superior and inferior ophthalmic veins. These in turn empty into a space called the cavernous sinus. This venous space is a vulnerable place because of all the structures that pass through it. The superior ophthalmic vein collects branches from some facial veins, making it possible for infections due to facial injuries to be communicated to the cavernous sinus. This sinus also has the internal carotid artery passing through it as well as some of the cranial nerves (see Chapter Nine), including the oculomotor, trochlear and ophthalmic nerves that have specific ocular functions. Also, the optic nerve and pituitary gland are adjacent to the cavernous sinus. One can easily appreciate that infection or disease of any of the structures in and around the cavernous sinus can result in ocular symptoms.

Ultimately, from the cavernous sinus, venous blood finds its way into the internal jugular vein, located in the neck. The internal jugular joins with the subclavian vein to form the brachiocephalic vein, the two of which (right and left) merge to form the superior vena cava, the short, wide vein that returns blood to the heart.

Now, to mirror the description of the arterial circulation, we return to the retina. To recap, the central retinal artery was described emerging from the within the optic nerve to branch out across the retina as ever-smaller vessels and ultimately capillaries. The retinal venous system travels much the same path in reverse, converging as the central retinal vein. At the smallest level, the capillaries and post-capillary veins are surrounded by a complicated and intricate system of cells and fibres. This structure was first properly described by Krückmann in 1917 after his examination of the retina of the freshly-injected head of a criminal immediately after his execution.

The central retinal vein exits the eye via the optic nerve, much as the central retinal artery enters it. After emerging from the optic nerve, it too drains into the cavernous sinus, either independently or via merging with the superior ophthalmic vein.

To end this chapter, it would be only right to mention another remarkable character who contributed so much to the understanding of the eye's anatomy. Niels Steensen (1638 – 86), sometimes known as Nicolaus Steno) was a Danish anatomist and fellow student of the aforementioned Frederik Ruysch at Leiden University. His interest to us is that he described the vortex veins (which were subsequently known as Steno's veins); but he also discovered the ducts that led him to conclude that the lacrimal gland was responsible for secreting tears, ending a controversy that extended back to the Greco-Roman physician Galen. And he discovered both 'Stensen's duct' that leads from the parotid gland into the mouth, and the follicles of the ovary. He also gave the first proper explanation of the structure of muscle and demonstrated that the heart is a muscle.

Not content with anatomy, he also made major contributions to palaeontology, crystallography and geology, within which field he is considered to be one of the founders of stratigraphy (the study of strata in rocks). Nevertheless, he left his post of Regius Professor of Anatomy at Copenhagen to convert from Lutheranism to Catholicism in Florence and become a priest. His work at the forefront of the counter-Reformation led to his beatification by Pope John Paul II in 1988.

CHAPTER NINE

THE EXTRA-OCULAR MUSCLES

'Joy in looking and comprehending is nature's most beautiful gift.' Albert Einstein

The muscles referred to in the title of this chapter are not optional extras; they are 'extra' in the sense of being outside the eye. These are the muscles mentioned briefly in the Introduction as being the ones that are responsible for moving the eyes around. For ease, the term 'extra-ocular' is often shortened to simply 'EO'.

It is impossible to talk properly about the EO muscles without also mentioning the nerves that supply them, since a problem with any of these nerves will affect the functioning of the relevant muscle(s) in ways that may be clearly visible to an observer. The Introduction also noted in passing the twelve cranial nerves and their importance to the eye. These are nerves that originate directly from the brain, as opposed to the spinal column. A quarter of these nerves are completely devoted to the eye muscles. Another, the optic nerve, is entirely concerned with vision. And a fifth (the Vth cranial, or trigeminal, nerve, as it happens) has one of its three branches - the ophthalmic nerve - supply various parts of the eye (along with some areas of

139

the nose) with sensory fibres. So, all in all, five of these twelve special nerves are concerned with the eye. It is not necessary to list all twelve here; they can be easily looked up in an anatomy text book. I am grateful to a fellow student and friend of mine who came up with an extremely rude mnemonic for remembering them, the very rudeness making it wonderfully effective as an *aide memoire* but, for obvious reasons, unrepeatable here.

What is important is to see the link between the EO muscles and their cranial nerves. It is also vital to know how each of the EO muscles moves the eyeball. To that end, below are shown two tables. Table 1 gives the names of the EO muscles together with the relevant name and number of the cranial nerve that supplies each one (the usual convention is to use Roman numerals for the nerves).

muscle	abbrev.	cranial nerve no.	cranial nerve name
Superior Rectus	SR	III	Oculo-motor
Inferior Rectus	IR	III	Oculo-motor
Medial Rectus	MR	III	Oculo-motor
Inferior Oblique	IO	III	Oculo-motor
Sup. Oblique	SO	IV	Trochlear
Lateral Rectus	LR	VI	Abducens

Table 1: The EO muscles and their cranial nerves

Table 2 lists the EO muscles with their main functions. Four of the six muscles (all, that is, except the medial and lateral recti) have additional functions that, in concert with other EO muscles, help execute all the possible movements of the eyeball within the orbit.

Muscle	Primary sphere of action on eyeball
SR	Upwards
IR	Downwards
MR	Inwards (towards nose)
LR	Outwards
SO	Inward rotation
IO	Outward rotation

Table 2: The EO muscles and their primary spheres of action

Let's Have a Look Around

None of the wonderful intricacies of visual perception would be of much use to us if we weren't able to direct our eyes accurately towards the desired object of attention. Furthermore, with two eyes in our heads, a mechanism for enabling them to act in concert is vital, otherwise double vision would result. Objects move across our field of vision;

we move through our environment. Objects move toward and away from us and vice versa. And what about the movements your eyes are making now, as you read this book, following the words across the page from left to right, then zooming back across the page to the start of the next line (or vice versa if you happen to be reading, say, a Hebrew translation)? With six muscles controlling each eye, the neurological systems involved in moving an eye to keep track of an object and co-ordinating these movements to exactly correlate with the other eye are, as can be imagined, incredibly complex. However, eye movements can broadly be divided into four categories:

- Smooth pursuit
- Vergence
- Saccades
- Vestibulo-ocular

Smooth pursuit movements are those that involve the eyes moving in the same direction as each other while tracking a moving object. These movements require a synergy of both nervous input to the relevant muscles of the two eyes, and reciprocal actions of pairs of muscles of each eye. As an example, imagine tracking an object moving from left to right horizontally across your field of vision. The most important muscles in allowing the eyes to follow that movement are the left MR / right LR pair. The MR of the left eye and the LR of the right eye must contract just sufficiently (and no more or less) to turn the two eyes rightwards at exactly the same rate. Pairs of muscles like this that move the eyes in the same direction in what are called *version* movements are called *yoke* muscles. Ewald Hering (1834 - 1918) proposed a law (that now bears his name) whereby each of the yoke muscles must receive an equal and simultaneous nervous input to achieve that movement.

Each of these two muscles has a muscle in its own eye that has the opposite function, known as an *antagonist*. The antagonist of the right LR is the right MR and, as the LR contracts, the MR must relax accordingly to effect the rightward turn of the eye. This is known as 'Sherrington's Law of reciprocal innervation' (nerve imput). Named after the noted English neurophysiologist and Nobel Prize winner Sir Charles Scott Sherrington (1857 – 1952), it states that when one muscle is stimulated, a muscle that works against the activity of the first will be inhibited. In other words, in order to make a simple left-to-right tracking movement, the brain has to co-ordinate the muscles of each eye in accordance with Sherington's Law and the muscles of the two eyes together in accordance with Hering's Law. That is complicated enough without considering that, in most version eye movements, other of the EO muscles will come into play, and all except the LR and MR muscles have secondary functions when the eye is in different positions; for instance, the SR, whose main function is upward movement, can act to rotate the eye inward in some circumstances.

Vergence eye movements are those that move the eyes in opposite directions in order to follow or focus on objects nearer (convergence) or further away (divergence). When one wants to focus on a near object, the accommodation required (see Chapter Six), creates a stimulus for the eyes to converge. This type of eye movement is, not surprisingly, called *accommodative convergence* (AC). The relationship between AC and accommodation, known as the 'AC/A ratio' is of great importance to the maintenance of binocular vision and is something that the optometrist pays much attention to when examining your eyes although you may not realise it.

Think for a moment of a hyperopic (long-sighted) person: they will have to work that extra bit hard to pull their focus in to view a near object compared with a non-hyperope. That extra accommodative effort induces greater AC. Sometimes, when the hypermetropia is of such a degree that it overtaxes the AC, the relationship breaks down and one or other eye converges too far, resulting in an inward-turning squint. It may be possible to correct the squint by correcting the hypermetropia with spectacles. The spectacles take care of the excess accommodative effort, so reducing the AC stimulus.

It can also be the case that someone who has had their vision uncorrected or under-corrected for some time finds that, on trying on their new spectacles containing the proper prescription, giving beautifully clear vision, there nevertheless results an uncomfortable 'pulling' or 'drawing' sensation of the eyes. This may be because they have learned to cope with an abnormal AC/A ratio, and those lovely new spectacles have interfered with that ratio. I should mention that there are all sorts of other reasons why new spectacles may feel uncomfortable, but consideration of the possible effects of a new or changed prescription on the AC/A ratio and other aspects of the visual system is part of the optometrist's prescribing skills.

Incidentally, the optometrist may turn the above scenario on its head in order to treat a patient who has difficulty converging. Prescribing spectacles that render the patient artificially slightly hyperopic can provide enough additional AC stimulus, through the extra accommodation required when using the spectacles, to overcome the problem. It supposes that the patient has sufficient facility of accommodation so, given that such facility decreases with age, the technique is more likely to be successful when applied to a younger person. This is but one more example for illustrative purposes, but there are many causes of binocular vision problems that can arise from a defective vergence system, unusually high or low AC/A ratio, defective EO muscles, abnormal nerve innervation to the muscles or any combination of these.

'Saccade' was the name originally applied to the rapid movements between pauses to fix on a word or phrase that occur when reading, but now refers to any rapid version movement of the eyes between fixation points. The term was apparently coined by the French ophthalmologist Louis Émile Javal (1839 – 1907), whose life it is worth making a short digression to outline. He initially qualified as a civil engineer; but his interest in eyes, due to his family's and his own ocular history, led him to study medicine and specialise in ophthalmology. His main interest was binocular vision and squints, although his name is probably most familiar to optometry students for his design, in collaboration with one of his students, Hjalmar Schiøtz, of an instrument to measure corneal curvature: the Javal Schiøtz keratometer.

Of interest to us here, he was the first to describe how eye movements during reading consisted of a series of rapid short movements (saccades) punctuated by stops (fixations). Sadly, Javal developed glaucoma in his right eye at the age of 45, eventually losing all vision by the time he was 62, leaving him blind for the last seven years of his life. This, despite unsuccessful surgery by an old English colleague and expert in the field, Priestly Smith. In a generous gesture, his wish after death was for cremation but that his left eye should be saved for research. It was duly removed and sent to Smith in Birmingham.

Saccades, rapid simultaneous movements of both eyes in the same direction, are actually the fastest movements that a human body can make. They can be triggered consciously when wishing to explore an environment, the eyes moving quickly from point to point. For instance, a trace can be made of saccadic eye movements made when looking at a face; the eyes will typically move from feature

146

to feature – eyes, nose, mouth – and around the outline of the face. Or, saccades can be part of consciously following the writing on a page, as described by Javal. Alternatively, saccades can result as a reflex reaction to a sudden appearance of a peripheral stimulus.

An interesting phenomenon of normal vision that combines both smooth pursuit and saccadic eye movements is *optokinetic nystagmus* (OKN). Nystagmus covers a range of involuntary oscillating eye movements, sometimes too small to see but often quite noticeable and most commonly horizontally, that can be pathological (congenital or acquired), or physiological. OKN, being a normal response to a moving, repeating stimulus, is the latter. The classic example is staring out of a train window watching telegraph poles go by. A smooth movement follows one pole and then the eyes flick back in a saccade in order to follow the next pole. The effect can be mimicked easily with the use of a rotating drum with vertical black and white stripes. Because OKN is a reflex action, the rotating drum set-up can be an effective, if basic, way of checking that an infant's visual system is intact; it can also be used as a way for ferreting out a malingerer who is feigning blindness.

A form of high-frequency physiological nystagmus is present constantly although you would not realise it, and it is essential for maintaining the 'picture' that you see when you are concentrating on an object. It sounds counter-intuitive that it should be necessary for the eyes to

147

wobble very quickly back and forth when you want to ex-amine something closely, but the reason this is so is due to the physiology of the retinal receptors. These receptors require constant fresh stimulation to keep firing and send-ing signals to the visual cortex, and the constant micro-movements of the eyes result in exactly that happening. Otherwise, the object of regard would gradually fade away. Thus physiological nystagmus moves the eyes less than one degree, ensuring that every point of the retinal image is moved by about the distance between two cones at the macula every tenth of a second or less even when you think you are staring fixedly at an object.

The final class of eye movement concerns the ves-tibulo-ocular reflex (VOR). Head movements require a re-sponse from the EO muscles in order for the eyes to retain fixation on a target; that extremely accurate response is provided by the VOR, which produces eye movements pre-cisely matching the degree of head movement but in the opposite direction.

The vestibular input is necessary for the VOR because it is sensory information provided by apparatus in the ears that gives us our sense of place and balance, co-ordinating motor movements to maintain these positional properties. The otolith organs, comprising the utricle and saccule lo-cated in the vestibule of the bony labyrinth of the inner ear are responsible for detecting linear motion and gravita-tional cues to position. The three semicircular canals de-tect rotational movements. The auditory-vestibular (or

148

vestibulocochlear) nerve, which is number VIII of the twelve cranial nerves, carries this information in its vestibular branch to the vestibular nucleus in the brain from where some neurons project to the EO muscle nuclei. If that vestibular input is impaired the eyes will tend to drift away from the perceived direction of motion, resulting in vertigo.

A form of the VOR, called the oculocephalic reflex, or 'Doll's Eyes' reflex, for reasons which will become clear in the following description, can be used to test for the presence of functioning brainstem eye movement pathways in the comatose patient. By holding the eyes open and moving the patient's head up and down and side to side, a reflex will be seen to be elicited if the eyes move in the opposite direction to those head movements.

A Turn for the Worse

We have looked at the EO muscle-related problems caused when vergence movements go awry due to a faulty relationship with the stimulus to accommodate (the AC/A ratio) which, in turn, often results from vision problems, especially high degrees of hypermetropia. Another type of vision error, *anisometropia*, where the error is very different between the eyes, can give rise to one eye becoming 'lazy', or *amblyopic*, which results in a lack of stimulus to the muscles of that eye to keep it moving in concert with the other eye. More directly, a problem with one of the cranial nerves that supplies the EO muscles will affect eye movements. This latter category is interesting for what it can tell us about what is going on in the brain, but it is a complex area because these nerves follow long and winding courses to their cranial origins, passing through and adjacent to many structures, any of which could acquire a pathological condition.

The end result of any disruption of the normal system of eye movements is that that eye will be turned inwards, outwards, upwards, downwards and, sometimes even obliquely with respect to the other eye. There are several terms for such a condition, ranging from, simply, 'a turn' in the eye, to the more clinical 'squint', 'strabismus' or 'tropia', to the old-fashioned 'cast'. For ease, I will stick with squint (although it should be mentioned that, used in this sense, the word has no relation to the act of squinting to see something by screwing the eyes up to peer at an object).

The accommodative squints and the ones due to errors of vision such as hypermetropia and anisometropia ('refractive' squints) generally develop in early childhood and will often be treated initially by methods that aim to correct the relevant type of error. This may be by prescribing spectacles, and/or covering the good eye for periods if the squinting eye already has reduced visual capacity (this harks back to the work of Hubel and Wiesel encountered in Chapter One) or initiating eye exercises. Sometimes, if an eye can't be straightened by these means, an operation is necessary to correct the squint. The two main options are muscle *resection* – removing a segment of an EO muscle in order to shorten it, thereby giving it effectively more 'pull'; and *recession*, whereby the insertion of the EO muscle into the eyeball is moved posteriorly, effectively reducing its 'pulling' power.

Squints acquired through injury or disease can, of course, happen at any time of life. The causes and manifestations are many, and it would take a whole textbook of ophthalmology to begin to do the sheer variety of them justice. It suffices here to summarise a few examples. Paresis, that is a partial or complete paralysis, of the oculomotor nerve (IIIrd cranial nerve) is one of the more common EO muscle problems encountered, due to its particularly long course from its nucleus in the brain and its consequent closeness to many important cranial structures. Although the oculomotor nerve supplies four of the EO muscles, the MR tends to be particularly affected by injury to it. So cranial tumours that press on the oculomotor nerve at any location can cause MR paresis; aneurysm of certain arteries that pass close to the nerve, likewise.

One of the more common causes of EO muscle palsy, especially of the LR or MR, is diabetes. A feature of diabetes is the shutting down of small vessels, or capillaries, which denies oxygen to the tissue that they supply. That is why the extremities - fingers and toes - are vulnerable to poor circulation in this disease. The oculomotor nerve is also vulnerable, but establishment of good diabetic control will often see the palsy resolve spontaneously after a few

151

weeks. It is distressing for a patient, though, because one of the early features of an acquired palsy is double vision.

Neuro-ophthalmology is all about having an intimate knowledge of the neural pathways that affect the eyes, looking for and eliciting the relevant ocular signs and deducing from them the affected pathway and likely site of its interruption. For instance, the oculomotor nerve supplies, in addition to four of the EO muscles, a major eyelid muscle as well as the sphincter muscle of the pupil; so a IIIrd nerve palsy can result in an outward (and downward) turned eye, a drooped eyelid and a dilated pupil. In fact, we saw some examples of this in the discussion of the pupil in Chapter Five.

There are two routine tests that an optometrist normally performs during an eye examination that relate to all of the above. They are quite simple and brief, so you may never have given them much thought. (Next time you have an eye examination, go on: *ask!* Any optometrist worth their salt should be happy to explain any part of the examination. Personally, I'm happy that you're taking an interest in what I'm doing.) The first of these tests involves covering one eye, removing the cover, covering the other eye and, again, removing the cover. This is called - wait for it – the 'cover test.' It is nothing to do with comparing the vision between the two eyes, which it probably seems like. Instead, the optometrist is looking for two types of movements of the eyes as the cover is placed and removed. The first type signifies a squint which, if too small to be seen by merely observing the eyes, may only be elicited by performing a cover test. If an eye is turned in, for instance, then when the other eye is covered it will move outwards to a 'straight' position to take up fixation of the object of regard. If it is turned out, it will move inwards when the other eye is covered, and so on.

The second type of movement shows the natural 'resting position' of the eyes, which gives clues to the status of the binocular system and factors like the AC/A ratio and the effect of the spectacle prescription on all of this. So, if the natural 'resting position' of the eyes is slightly out then, on removing the cover from an eye, that eye will move inwards to straight ahead from its natural position, to join the other eye in fixating an object. If the natural position is inward, the eye moves outwards on being uncovered. The degree of movement can be different when the eyes are fixing a far or near object, so the test is usually repeated for both situations. These movements can be extremely subtle, but an experienced observer can glean a lot of information from a test that takes perhaps less than half a minute.

The second test referred to above aims to check that the workings of the EO muscles are in order. Again, on the surface, it is a very simple, quick, test. But it can provide clues to many of the EO muscle problems already described. In the 'ocular motility' test, the patient is asked to look at a hand-held target and asked to follow it as it is moved up, down, left, right and along both diagonals. This gives an overview of the movements of the EO muscles in their primary positions of action. The two eyes should move equally and in concert. Any discrepancy in the eyes' movements or report from the patient of doubling of the target in any position suggests a weakness for whatever reason in one (or more) of the EO muscles. The direction in which this discrepancy occurs provides the clue to the affected muscle.

Six muscles, several nerves, reflexes, various control and feedback mechanisms involving different parts of the brain: these are some of the vital 'backroom' functions that help us to see. The EO muscles are not strictly parts of the eye, although they are physically attached to the eyeball. But without them the eye would be just a highly complex, beautifully constructed, but useless, sphere of tissue.

CHAPTER TEN

COLOUR VISION

'All colours will agree in the dark.' Francis Bacon

'What colour is it? may seem a simple enough question. But, oh, what a can of worms is opened by that innocent query. Can an object even be said to have an intrinsic colour? Would two people with 'normal' colour vision perceive the same colour when looking at an object?

The answers to these questions, and others concerning the nature of colour vision, require us to examine the very nature of light, as argued over by physicists for centuries. We will accompany physiologists towards an explanation of how our perception of colour alters according to surrounding brightness; look in on physicists and lighting engineers to see how artificial lighting affects colour perception; and monitor the spat among all and sundry as to the correct description of the mechanism of colour vision. We'll also find out what happens when that mechanism (whatever it is) is faulty, and how we can assess the extent of the problem. Excuse the obvious pun approaching, but the subject of colour vision is far from black and white.

Let's start by trying to get to grips with this: what is light? In the seventeenth century Sir Isaac Newton and Robert Hooke had a long-running bitter argument about just that, mediated by Henry Oldenberg, secretary for correspondence at the Royal Society. What is interesting about the dispute is that each of the protagonists had reached his conclusions as a result of the outcome of his own, seemingly conclusive, experiments; it was no idle slanging-match about unsubstantiated theories.

Newton (1642 - 1727) is the last, and perhaps most famous, of the Lucasian professors of mathematics whom we shall meet. He came to the chair aged only 26. His work on light, colour and optics occupied a large proportion of his career, but he only published it, in *Opticks*, in 1706, when he realised that others were making similar findings and might get the credit for them.

Newton's experiments in 1666, reported to Oldenberg in 1672, involved the production of a spectrum by passing light from a gap in his shuttered windows through a prism, to be projected on to the wall opposite. At first, due to the fact that the beam of light passing through the prism was deflected or, more properly, refracted, Newton wondered whether the action of the prism was to make the light rays move in a curved path. He refined his experiments to enable him to look for likely effects of curved motion but found none. It was clear that light travelled in straight lines and he concluded that light consists of rays of particles, white light being a mixture of rays tending to different amounts of refraction when passed through a medium such as glass. These differing amounts of refraction produced the colours of the spectrum that he saw via his prism.

His calculations on the spread of 'refractance' across the spectrum led him to a depressing realisation about the ultimate quality of the image obtainable from optical lenses - especially those used in optical telescopes. Newton realised that however well a lens focused on one part of the spectrum, the other parts would be out of focus; in other words, in collecting white light, a lens would inevitably separate out some colours - what we would call chromatic aberration.

He speculated on the use instead of a mirror to collect light for a telescope, with a parabolic shape to focus the light to a point. Indeed, he eventually built a reflecting telescope of much-improved performance over what was then available. However, his opponent Hooke also built a reflecting telescope – in 1664, probably three or four years before Newton constructed his first.

Hooke (1635 - 1703) initially showed aptitude in painting and was sent to London to be tutored by Sir Peter Lely. A master at Westminster School recognised his intellectual potential and, under his guidance, Hooke gained a place at Christ Church, Oxford. As gregarious as Newton was introverted, he became assistant to Robert Boyle, who secured for him the post of Curator of Experiments at the newly-formed Royal Society. His interests led him to theo-

157

ries of mechanics, gravity and optics, as well as hypotheses in subjects as diverse as botany, anatomy, geology, cartography, telescopes, engines and microscopes. His greatest work, *Micrographia* (1665), was a treatise on microscopy, but also contained some original theories on the nature of light. The scene was set for a bitter rivalry which endured until Hooke's death.

Hooke's reply to Newton's letter to Oldenberg was polite, if a little condescending to Newton. He stressed the hundreds of experiments he had performed which led him to the conclusion that light is made up of pulses, or waves; and that colour arises from the disturbances of these waves when passing through another transparent medium. Newton then made his own reply, stating why he felt that light could not possibly be a wave. Each correspondent felt that his own theory was sufficient to explain the other's results. And here's the supreme irony: they were both right!

Classic experiments, such as Thomas Young's in 1801, demonstrated diffraction and interference of light - both properties of waves. Not until nearly a hundred years later did the tide begin to turn. Experimental evidence was now being accumulated for which the wave theory of light could not offer a proper explanation. Based on the ideas of Max Planck, Albert Einstein (1879 - 1955) formulated an equation that suggested light travels in discrete packets, or particles, called photons. Further experiments have since confirmed the validity of Einstein's equation. Light is now considered to exhibit 'wave-particle duality'.

There is a further irony, in a way, given that Newton's experiments with prism spectra were instrumental in his forming a particle theory of light, in that colour is most commonly described in terms of wavelength. When light is passed through a prism the beam is bent in a precise way, which is described by *Snell's Law*. The amount of bending is in roughly inverse proportion to the wavelength of the light; so short wavelengths (blue light) are bent more than long wavelengths (red). The narrow beam is thus split up and displayed in its component colours.

It is important to realise that the colours which make up visible light are just a small part of the range of the electromagnetic radiation spectrum. There is nothing special about them, it's just that our eyes, as optical instruments, are only capable of detecting those wavelengths - which, by definition, we call visible. The names of other parts of the electromagnetic spectrum arise from the way we detect or use them, such as microwaves or radio waves. 'Colour' is really only a human sensory construct. From a physical viewpoint we can say that blue light is just that electromagnetic radiation with a wavelength of around 0.46µm, but its 'blueness' only exists as our *perception* of it as such.

Perception is the key word. The eye is designed to collect useful amounts of electromagnetic radiation within a range of wavelengths. This is only of real use if the visual system is able to process the information to a level that can discriminate between these wavelengths. And, of course, it can, delivering the data in such a way that the brain perceives the various wavelengths as a range of colours. If you are ahead of me, you are already wondering how the visual apparatus achieves such a colour-discriminating system. This question leads the way to the battleground of the next section.

Component or Opponent?

Step forward our next protagonists. In one corner we have the decipherer of the Rosetta Stone, and the descendant of the founder of Pennsylvania: Thomas Young and Hermann von Helmholtz, with both of whom we are familiar. In the opposite corner, stand up professor of Physiology at Prague, Ewald Hering, who we met in the last chapter. If the line-ups appear a little one-sided, they seem more unbalanced when we find that another player has to be added to the Young-Helmholtz partnership. He is James Clerk Maxwell (1831 - 79), a Scot, and first Cavendish professor of Experimental Physics at Cambridge University.

Maxwell is another figure who has had an enormous impact on several areas of physics, not least the kinetic theory of gases, the theoretical nature of Saturn's rings (later confirmed) and, of course, colour perception. He even demonstrated colour photography by taking a picture of a tartan ribbon. He is best known, though, for his work on electromagnetic waves; his *Treatise on Electricity and*

Magnetism, published in 1873, put the work of the great Michael Faraday into mathematical terms and laid the foundation for the theories of Einstein and Planck. Not bad for a lad nicknamed 'Dafty' at school.

Could Hering hold his end up against such distinguished opposition? We shall see.

Young was first off the mark. In 1801 he gave the Bakerian lecture at the Royal Society (later published in 1802) in which he set out the basic ideas of what was to become known as the *trichromatic theory* of colour vision. Subsequent modifications came from Helmholtz, notably in 1866 and 1896, while much work was added by Maxwell in the latter half of the century. As a result the trichromatic, or *component*, theory is often referred to as the Young-Helmholtz-Maxwell theory.

What Young suggested in his lecture was this:

'Now, as it is almost impossible to conceive each sensitive point of the retina to contain an infinite number of particles, each capable of vibrating in perfect unison with every possible undulation, it becomes necessary to suppose the number limited, for instance, to the three principal colours, red, yellow and blue.'

Helmholtz and Maxwell gathered experimental evidence to support this idea by showing that human colour perception could be best described by a system of three primary colours which, in varying proportions, produced normal colour responses. This could be achieved in the visual system in one of three ways: having three photochemicals in the cones sensitive to different wavelengths of light; or the presence of three different cone types; or three different nerve fibre pathways.

Hering's observations of colour appearances led him to believe that the trichromatic theory was not sufficient to explain the mixing of colours to produce another colour or a colourless sensation. Some pairs of colours seemed not to mix at all, but to produce an appearance of white. That is to say they are mutually exclusive; for instance, one would never see a colour that could be described as reddish-green or bluish-yellow.

In 1875 Hering proposed his *opponent theory* of colour vision which suggested that there are three pairs of colour processes present in the visual system and that members of each pair oppose one another. These pairs are: red-green, blue-yellow and black-white. By this way of thinking white is not a 'combined' colour sensation, but a single, direct experience. Hering's theory was largely neglected until the work of two researchers, Hurvich and Jameson, in the early 1970s.

Thus far all that could be said on the subject was hypothetical, backed up by some experimental evidence on each side. Maxwell did much to put Helmholtz's work on finding combinations of three colours to produce the same colour sensations as a reference light, on a mathematical footing. Arguments about the validity of each theory were

162

especially intense, since it was assumed that the correctness of one theory precluded the other - much as with Newton's and Hooke's dispute over the nature of light. And nothing at all had been said yet to suggest where exactly the anatomical and physiological apparatus that each theory predicted was located.

Not until the middle of the twentieth century did the first evidence of this nature begin to accumulate. The new technique of microspectrophotometry enabled studies to be made of individual photoreceptors in the retina. Three distinct classes of cones were identified, each having different, but overlapping, wavelength sensitivities. They are casually referred to as blue, green and red cones due to their respective maximum sensitivities at those parts of the spectrum.

Generally speaking, since the overall sensitivities of each type of cone overlap, a stimulation of the retina by a single wavelength of light will cause a combined stimulation (of differing proportions) of all three cone types. The ascendancy of the trichromatic theory of Young, Helmholtz and Maxwell seemed assured.

Another technique for investigating the visual system, electrophysiology, was by now well-established. In fact, the first electrophysiological work in investigating vision was initiated by DuBois Reymund in 1849, when he managed to measure the electrical activity within the eye. With the advent of electronic amplification, electrical responses could be obtained from individual retinal elements using micro-electrodes.

The record of electrical activity generated in the retina in response to light stimulation is called the electroretinogram (ERG); the first ERG was obtained in 1903. When the rod and cone photoreceptors are stimulated, they send signals along a chain of neurones to nerve cells called ganglion cells. Many photoreceptor signals are routed to one ganglion cell. And it is the ganglion cell signal, the result of processing many photoreceptor responses, that is sent via the optic nerve to the brain. Thus the realisation by the 1950s that photoreceptors do not act independently of each other.

By the 1970s much work had been focused on these ganglion cells. At least eleven different types had been delineated. Importantly for our discussion of colour vision it was found that these different types of cell could be identified as belonging to one of two systems, depending on their function. And one system could be divided into three distinct sub-systems which are related to the red, green and blue mechanisms.

The cells in these sub-groups are served by several cones (known as the cell's receptive field), the cone-type sending the strongest signal determining whether the ganglion cell will pass a signal on. Since a cell's receptive field receives signals from two cone-types, say red and green, there is an *opponent* system operating. At last Hering's general idea was vindicated.

164

But haven't we already shown that the trichromatic theory is correct? Only up to a point, as it does not explain all the features of colour vision satisfactorily. The best and fullest description of the mechanism of colour vision is arrived at, ultimately, by thinking of the two theories, trichromatic and opponent, as complementary rather than mutually exclusive. This is reminiscent of the Newton-Hooke dispute; each theory describes different but complimentary aspects of the same phenomenon.

It is generally accepted now that the trichromatic theory best describes events at the photoreceptor level, where there are indeed three kinds of cone, each with a peak sensitivity to a particular colour (red, green, blue). The opponent theory, meanwhile, gives a better sense of what has been discovered about the neural processes; how the nerve signals at various points in the visual pathway are encoded so that information about colour can be interpreted by the brain. And what a fascinatingly complicated coding mechanism it is - but, alas, beyond the scope of this book.

The Red (and Green) Mist

Colour-blindness. An emotive phrase, but what does it actually mean? If one were truly blind to colour, the world would appear to exist only in black and white. Clearly this is not the case for most colour-blind people, although the condition does, rarely, occur. Most affected people can see a wide range of colours but find it difficult to distinguish shades from among specific groups of colours. More properly such people nowadays are referred to as colour-deficient. An alternative label is Daltonism, after the man who first described the condition in detail.

John Dalton (1766 - 1844) was born near Cockermouth in Cumbria, the son of a Quaker weaver. He developed a love of scientific studies during his joint proprietorship, with his brother, of a boarding-school. In 1787 he started a meteorological journal which eventually was to include 200,000 observations. He became, in 1793, a mathematics and science teacher at New College, Manchester and, in 1794, he first described colour-deficiency - as suffered by his brother and himself. Thanks to his chemical and physical studies, he has an eponymous law of gases - *Dalton's Law of Partial Pressures* - to add to the Daltonism of colour-deficiency.

Colour-deficiency takes several forms and has almost infinite gradations of severity. The most common forms are hereditary, via female carriers. The inherited genetic defect causes an absence or defect in one or more of the cone photopigments. The condition affects approximately 8 per cent of the male population and around 0.5 per cent of females.

Consider, for a moment, what that figure of 8 per cent for males means in terms of, say, a football match. Statistically at least one player out of the twenty-two on the pitch is likely to be colour-defective. Not only may he have a problem distinguishing between the teams' colours, he may find one of the colours more difficult to pick out from the background of the crowd. Factor in the penchant of some teams (eg England, Manchester United) to play in grey and, for the reasons explained presently, his problems are multiplied.

Let's clarify the classification of colour defects further: normal colour vision, dependent on three types of cone pigment, is termed *trichromatism.* One or more defective photopigments results in *anomalous trichromatism.* The complete absence of one photopigment causes *dichromatism*; other terms are introduced to specify whether the faulty mechanism is red, green or blue. Alteration in colour perception can arise through injury or disease. These acquired forms of colour defect are often termed *dyschromatopsias.*

Those of us with normal colour perception have the amazing ability to distinguish among wavelengths of light corresponding to over a hundred different hues within the visible spectrum. The colour-deficient tend to confuse groups of colours such as reds, browns, oranges, yellows and greens because they appear indistinguishable from each other. More precisely, those dichromats missing the red-sensitive cones have, not surprisingly, a reduced perception of the red end of the spectrum; and the blue-green part of the spectrum appears grey. The green-missing dichromats have a grey area in the normal green part of the spectrum.

In the more common case of anomalous trichromatism, where one or more of the cone mechanisms is merely defective, the grey areas give way to zones of indistinct, or washed-out, colours. To summarise, for those with red-green deficiencies (by far the most common) blues and yellows generally seem clearer and more distinct than reds and greens.

How Green is My Green?

Modern tests for colour vision make use of the areas of colour confusion experienced by colour defectives by incorporating carefully chosen colour combinations. It was not always so. The first recorded colour vision test was introduced in Sweden in 1876 as a result of a major rail crash in which a misreading of signals was implicated. The test comprised skeins of wool of varying colour and brightness, from which samples had to be chosen that matched each of four control wools coloured red, green, grey and purple.

So-called trade or vocational tests were gradually developed, some of which are in use today. These rely on reproducing the actual working conditions under which colours need to be distinguished. The train drivers' lantern test is a prime example: lights such as those used in signals are presented in a strictly defined sequence, which the candidate is asked to identify. Alternatively, an electrician may be asked to name various colour-coded resistors and wires.

A more detailed scientific analysis of vision can be made using something called the Farnsworth-Munsell 100-Hue test. The 100-Hue test examines the ability to tell similar colours apart, across the whole of the colour spectrum. The modern version actually only has 85 hues - it was reduced from 100 by Farnsworth - of precise specifications reproduced on a particular type of paper: Munsell paper; hence the name of the test. The subject is asked to place caps containing the coloured papers in strict order of closeness of hue to each preceding cap. The caps are all numbered so that the subject's attempt can be plotted easily on a circular chart. Even a colour-normal subject is likely to make a few mistakes so the circular plot, representing error scores, will be a roughly circular graph line with one or two outward spikes representing the mistakes.

A colour-deficient subject, however, who will confuse certain groups of colours, will have a plot distinguished by huge spikes like solar flares at characteristic points on opposite sides of the circle. The size and position of these spikes help to determine the nature of the defect. The 100-Hue test is still in widespread use in hospitals, where it is used particularly to quantify acquired defects.

No discussion of colour vision tests would be complete - even though this is not an exhaustive survey - without mentioning the test devised by an emeritus professor of the University of Tokyo and member of the Japan Academy, one Dr. Shinobu Ishihara. Most people will be familiar with the Ishihara Pseudo-Isochromatic Plates (if not by name!). 'Pseudo-isochromatic' is a nice long term for colours which are different but appear the same under certain circumstances. The test comprises a number of plates each made up of patterns of differently coloured spots. Within the background, which comprises spots of mainly one hue, can be seen a one- or two-digit numeral formed by spots of another hue. The colour combinations are chosen carefully to fall within the confusion zones of the various types of colour defect.

Numbers which are discerned easily by a colour-normal subject will be read by a colour-deficient either as a specific, different number, or not seen at all. It is quite fascinating, as a colour-normal, to watch a colour-defective subject run through the Ishihara test blithely calling out all the 'wrong' answers; only to be dumbfounded when confronted with the 'correct' responses. I daresay Dr Ishihara was quite amused.

Blue Moon

We have covered only part of the colour story by discussing the mechanisms in the eye and visual system by which colours are detected and distinguished. Other factors come in to play that determine how the colour of an object is perceived. Some are due to the eye itself, others due to the quirks of the processing of visual information and still others to the physical characteristics of light sources.

If one measures the relative sensitivity of the eye to different wavelengths in the visible spectrum, under normal daytime illumination a curve is obtained which has a peak at around $0.555\mu m$ (corresponding to a yellowish-green colour) and then drops away on either side, towards red and blue. Johannes Purkinje, in yet another of his optical investigations, noticed something odd when illumination was decreased sufficiently. He described, in 1825, an effect whereby the peak of the curve described above shifted towards the blue end of the spectrum (to 0.505μm; a bluish-green colour) in poor light.

This change in the colour sensitivity of the eye is still known as the Purkinje Shift, so: having asked you to remember Purkinje when you see his 'tree' on having a light shone in your eye during an eye examination, I now ask you to step outside at dusk and, with Purkinje in mind, marvel at the enhanced blues and violets you see in your garden.

The Purkinje Shift is explained by the dual nature of the eye's visual system. During daytime, the eye's pupil being small, vision is largely mediated by the central area of the retina which is rich in colour-receptive cones, but which also contains a yellow pigment that absorbs blue light. At night, the blue-absorbing, cone-rich centre gives way in dominance to the rod-rich peripheral retina. You may have noticed, perhaps while driving, that during the period of dusk, before night has properly drawn in - what W B Yeats poetically called the half-light - that more concentration is required than in light or dark conditions. In this instance, the eye is at a halfway house, hovering between the light- and dark-adapted cone and rod systems where neither is working maximally.

Many strange colour and, more generally, light adaption effects have been described which are attributed to the processing of visual information. There are all sorts of stimulatory, inhibitory and feedback systems involved in visual processing, that can be likened to electronic control systems in engineering technology.

In the right conditions, one can demonstrate an after-image effect with colours. If an object of one colour is viewed for a period of time and then the gaze is switched, preferably, to a white background, a faint after-image of the complimentary colour may be seen, if only briefly. I shall mention only two other interesting effects. Neither is strictly a colour effect, but both arise from inhibitory processes in the visual system; and both are easy to see for yourself.

The first effect is called the Hering-Hermann grid. You need to find someone who has dark square tiles in their bathroom - with expertly executed white grouting. If you look at the grouting at an intersection between the corners of four tiles, you should become aware of darkened patches at all the surrounding white intersections. The whiter and wider the grouting and the darker the tiles the better. But don't spend too long in the bathroom on Hering's and Hermann's account.

On the other hand, perhaps linger long enough to appreciate the second effect, which is due to Ernst Mach (he of the speed of sound). Take two tiles of the same colour, except that one is of a darker shade than the other. Placed next to each other, with the border between them clearly defined, what should appear is a dark band on the dark-tile side of the border and a light band on the light-tile side. This is due to a sort of inhibitory over-compensation effect; the part of the dark tile next to the border seems darker because it is in immediate contrast with the light tile, and vice-versa for the light tile. It is possible to plot a graph comparing the subjective as against actual luminance of such a target. Then again, it's just fun to look at. Thank goodness, given all of these strange effects, for nice bright artificial lighting under which colours appear crisp and clear. Sorry, but no. This is straying somewhat away from the subject of eyes, but lighting does affect the way we perceive colour; and don't advertisers, marketers and interior designers know it. My bugbear is clothes shops: trying to work out exactly what colour a particular tie or jacket is can be a nightmare. Surely, I can't be the only person who has to pick up an item of clothing, turn it this way and that to catch it in the best light, and still find, when I get it home that it's not the colour I thought it was? Why is this - and why do shops do it?

Without wishing to scare off physics-phobes it is largely to do with two properties of light sources: colour rendering and colour appearance. Colour rendering is the term applied to the apparent colour of an object under any light source as compared with a standardised source such as daylight. (Of course, daylight can vary widely, but an agreed measure of brightness of averagely overcast northern sky is usually used.) Put rather simplistically, those sources that emit light strongly in one band of colour will have poor colour matching properties compared with one that emits a broad band of wavelengths of similar composition to daylight. This is what the designers want!

Come with me to the supermarket for the classic example. First, we'll visit the fruit and veg. Don't the vegetables all look beautifully green and fresh? Now we'll pass along to the meat counter. Look at all those red, succulent cuts. I would not wish to suggest that there is anything wrong with supermarket food, but the greenness of the vegetables is certainly helped along by being under a light source that emits strongly in the green part of the spectrum while different, reddish-dominant, lighting is used over at the meat counter to enhance its display.

Colour appearance, meanwhile, concerns the colour a light source itself appears to be (or a white surface seen by its light). Thus, lighting is often described as cool because it has a bluish tinge, or warm, due to its reddish hue. Warm lighting is used in many places to create an atmosphere of calm and relaxation.

Next time you are in the supermarket and your hackles are rising as a result of the latest price rise or ankle dig from a passing trolley, take a wander over to the meat section and bask in its calming pinkish-red glow for a few minutes. If you get some odd stares, it's only people wondering what it is that you're embarrassed about: under this colour rendering you may appear to be blushing.

174

CHAPTER ELEVEN

THE VISUAL PATHWAY

'... we are supposing the brain to be much more than a tel-ephone exchange'" Charles Scott Sherrington

Thus far we have travelled more or less methodically from the front of the eye to the back. The optic nerve forms part of the eye in that it is structurally connected to it and is the 'cable' which carries nerve fibres and the major blood vessels to and from the eye. It is also part of the visual pathway that is intimately connected with and, indeed, forms part of, the brain. So, we have come full circle: I mentioned right at the beginning of Chapter One that the eyes are direct outgrowths of the brain. To recap, the eyes develop as buds on the end of stalks comprised of embryonic brain material; these stalks become the optic nerves.

At this point, perhaps I should debunk a widely-held piece of 'common knowledge' and, in doing so, probably settle a few arguments. Consider the story told many a time by persons who have undergone an eye operation: 'It was amazing,' they say. 'The surgeon took my eye right out. I know that's what happened because I could feel my eyeball, cold and wet, resting on my cheek.' Oh, for the

175

proverbial pound for each time I have heard this story or something similar. Usually I raise an eyebrow as non-confrontationally as possible and move on quickly. I don't make a big thing of it, because the belief that it truly happened seems always to be held with such conviction that no amount of effort expended in arguing otherwise will shake that person's conviction. But that conviction is false! I repeat, false.

So what does happen during eye operations? Whatever the procedure, an eye is never to be found lolling about on the cheek like those joke spectacles with eyeballs on springs. Firstly, the optic nerve is not some springy or elastic extension cable. Secondly, there is just too much stuff packed into the eye socket and too many things attached to the eyeball to allow for much forward movement. This has been alluded to in respect of the conjunctiva in Chapter Two, but we will now delve more deeply into the contents of the bony orifice that houses the eye.

The Orbit

The eye socket, or orbit, is a roundish cavern at the front of the skull around 40mm deep and wide. At the back of the orbit are some small holes, or *foramina*, which allow various nerves and blood vessels to pass through into it. One of these holes, the *optic foramen*, is where the optic nerve passes into the orbit. Note, as mentioned above, that the optic nerve is not elastic and under compression just waiting for someone to release the eye from the orbit so that it can spring forward like a bungee rope.

Apart from the eyeball itself (a fairly tight fit anyway), the orbit houses the six extra-ocular muscles that enable the eye to move in different directions. At one end each muscle is inserted into the outer eyeball; at the other they come together to merge into what is called the *tendinous origin of Zinn* (he of the zonules), which attaches to the rear of the orbit. This arrangement, as well as the various nerves and blood vessels that enter the orbit through the foramina, not to mention the packing of orbital fatty tissue that fills any spare space, gives a pretty good picture of why the eyeball cannot just 'pop out'.

During an eye operation, it may be necessary for the surgeon to turn the eyeball into different positions (although in many procedures, for instance cataract removal, the eye needs to be kept still). How can this be achieved when the patient is under a general anaesthetic? The surgeon can hardly say to the slumbering patient, 'Look up please. Now look to your left.' In fact, if the eyelids are retracted sufficiently, enough of the eyeball can be exposed so that the eye muscle attachments to the eyeball can be seen. It is then relatively easy to isolate each muscle so that one or other of them can be made to move the eye in the desired direction. Forgive the (hopefully interesting) digression, but it serves to reinforce the fact that the eye is not like some rubber ball on the end of a piece of (optic nerve) elastic. It is such a strong myth, that the reality is worth emphasising.

A Window to the Brain

Functionally, the optic nerve begins in the retina, at the level of the ganglion cells. These feed the electrical signals - created by the rods and cones in response to light stimuli – into nerve fibres. From all across the retina these nerve fibres converge at the optic nerve. Pressure on the optic nerve in glaucoma (see Chapter Four) causes damage to bundles of these fibres, resulting in specific defects of the field of vision relating to the segments of the retina that these bundles originate from. As mentioned in Chapter Four, this damage occurs because the optic nerve is a weak spot in the wall of the eye. Why the weakness?

Most of the wall of the eyeball is made up of tough, opaque sclera or almost equally tough, transparent cornea. But there has to be a gap in the sclera to enable the nerve fibres within the optic nerve to pass into the eye. Two major blood vessels, the central retinal artery and central retinal vein, are also contained within the optic nerve at this point (they enter and exit the optic nerve just behind the eyeball). But rather than there being a simple hole into which the optic nerve is simply plugged, which would be an extremely weak arrangement, there is a dense meshwork of connective tissue across the entry point through whose gaps the components within the optic nerve can pass. This 'cribriform plate', or *lamina cribrosa*, has the twofold function of giving support to those components and minimising the potential weakness of the region.

The whole complex arrangement can be seen head-on when looking into the eye with an ophthalmoscope. In fact, it is one of the elements of the internal eye examination to which the optometrist will pay most attention, since any changes in the appearance of the head of the optic nerve (usually referred to as the optic disc) can be indicative of disease. From the pinkish oval of the optic disc can be seen emerging the superior and inferior branches of the retinal artery and vein. The disc, in most people, has a natural shallow depression within it. If the depression, or optic cup, is unusually large or deep compared with the norm or the fellow eye; or if the course of the emerging blood vessels seems altered; or the colour of the disc is unusually pale, these could all be signs of glaucoma.

A pale disc could also be a sign of damage or death of optic nerve fibres for a whole variety of other reasons, such as toxins (for example, chronic alcohol poisoning), injury or disease (for example, multiple sclerosis). Incidentally, why does multiple sclerosis (MS) affect vision in some sufferers? MS is what is known as a demyelinating disease. Most nerve fibres have a sheath of fatty tissue called myelin. This sheath acts as an insulator and helps the electrical signal to travel efficiently along the length of the nerve fibre. Without the sheath, some of the signal in effect 'leaks' away and so is conducted more slowly. The optic nerve fibres are just the same, so it is easy to imagine

179

the interruption caused to the processing of visual information that is sometimes caused in MS.

In some cases, on examination, the optic disc may appear to be swollen. Instead of a nice sharply-defined oval, the disc will have a blurred margin and distorted features (imagine looking down on a fluffed-up Spanish omelette in comparison with a flat pancake). Fortunately, it is a fairly rare occurrence but, when seen, can be of serious significance. Remember that the optic nerve has to travel from the eye right through the brain to the visual centre at the posterior (occipital) lobe. As it does so, it passes close by many important structures and blood vessels; so a problem with any of these can compress the optic nerve at that point. This then results in the swelling that is seen at the optic disc.

Worryingly for the optometrist, the severity of the patient's symptoms in such cases can be completely out of proportion to the seriousness of the cause. From personal experience I can recall seeing two cases in twenty-five years - both young adults and non-spectacle-wearers – presenting with grossly swollen optic discs. One had been experiencing unbearable thumping headaches for two days such that she couldn't even lie down to sleep. The other was vaguely concerned that occasionally, over the past few months, he had had the odd slight headache and thought he might need spectacles. It turned out that the first patient had raised cerebro-spinal fluid pressure – serious enough, but easily treated with no lasting damage;

the second had a tumour the size of a golf ball that was removed a few days later, which could have killed him within a few weeks.

The Eye-Brain Connection

We can think of the visual pathway as having seven distinct sections, of which the optic nerve is just one, joined together somewhat like elements of an electrical circuit. The fascination is in how all of these elements combine to produce a picture of the world around us and how, when things go wrong, we are able to use this knowledge to deduce what and where the problem is. A complete explanation of the visual process is even more complex, involving higher processing of visual information in many other centres of the brain, but the first priority is to get the raw information from the signal detected in the retina to the visual cortex where a basic visual picture emerges. The sections are:

1. Retina
2. Optic nerve
3. Optic chiasma
4. Optic tract
5. Lateral geniculate body
6. Optic radiation
7. Visual cortex

The retina, we have seen, acts as a transducer that converts energy in the form of light photons into electrical signals. A photon hitting the photosensitive retina sets of a cascade of biochemical reactions which in turn produce the electrical output. This converted sensory signal is led, via a complex pathway of retinal cells, to a final route beginning with the retinal ganglion cells. These ganglion cells are the only cells that connect directly from the eye to the brain, with most terminating at the lateral geniculate body. Hold tight: because we are now off and running to keep up with our nerve impulse.

Around a million nerve fibres are bundled into the optic nerve, which leaves the orbit via the optic foramen. To use the word 'bundled' is a little unfair, as the fibres are arranged in a precise way in the body of the nerve. Around a third of all the fibres relate to that tiny central area of the retina, the macula, which is responsible for much of the detail (and colour) of what we see. The other two-thirds carry signals from the remainder of the retina. We are moving rapidly towards the optic chiasma, the Clapham Junction of the visual pathway.

At this point we need to remind ourselves that the image of the outside world produced on the retina is inverted; that is, upside-down and back-to-front. This is due to the optical properties of the eye's focusing apparatus - looking through a convex lens at a fairly distant object will produce the same result (try borrowing someone's reading glasses to experiment with). Here's where the visual system employs a neat trick.

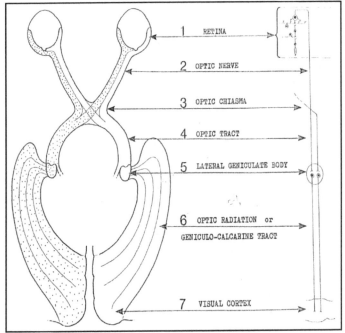

Figure 5. The visual pathway.

At the chiasma all the fibres from the nasal (inner) retina cross over to the opposite visual pathway to join with the temporal (outer) fibres from the other eye. If we take the nasal fibres from the right eye, these relate to the temporal (outer) or right-half of the picture that the right eye sees. Now add these to the temporal fibres from the left eye. These relate to the nasal (inner) or right-half of the picture that the left eye sees. So we have a situation where, after the chiasma, all the fibres from both eyes that relate to the right-half of our visual field are in the left optic tract and all those relating to the left visual field are in the right optic tract. Not only can we now see how the visual system cleverly creates a correct, right-way-round image of the world around us, but we also see how the general rule of sensory representation in the cerebral cortex of right side represented in the left hemisphere and vice versa is preserved.

The lateral geniculate body (LGB) is often considered as being merely a junction box; a relay station between nerve fibres carrying signals from the retina, and fibres transporting these signals to the visual cortex. The minute anatomy of the LGB, however, suggests that it has a processing role too. Remember that the signals from around 137 million rods and cones are sent up the optic nerve via only about one million nerve fibres - which suggests some processing occurs at the retinal level. The ratio of optic nerve fibres to LGB neurones is about 1:2. In other words, each LGB neurone has an average of two (or more) optic nerve fibres linked to it, each of which need to send signals for it to be stimulated.

This introduces the idea of *receptive fields*, which is important also when we consider the visual cortex. Extensive experimentation has shown that ultimately what stimulates the visual cortex are shapes, movement and borders between areas of different brightness and colour. Groups of retinal cells wired together form receptive fields for these attributes and the information is sent to LGB neurons which respond to each type of receptive field. The stimuli from these neurons are then forwarded, via the optic radiation, to the visual cortex. The cortical cells refine all of this information. Think about it for a moment: what sort of information is most useful to our visual system? It's anything to do with *change* in our surroundings such as movement and changes of shape, brightness and colour. A field of view that is completely static and unchanging is of little interest to us – because it will be just the same next time we look. What we really need to be aware of is anything (or anyone) moving or changing within our view. This may be because we want to find our way around our environment or because we need to be aware of potential predators or prey. By concentrating on these attributes of our environment, the visual system is able to filter out an enormous mass of irrelevant visual information that our eyes receive.

A footnote: suppose you were sitting completely still in a completely static environment. Would everything just fade to grey as the visual cortex stops being stimulated? In theory, yes! Fortunately, there is the clever mechanism of physiological nystagmus (referred to in Chapter Nine) whereby, even when the eyes are apparently still, there is a nervous input to the eye muscles that produces a series of constant tiny eye movements. So the visual picture is regularly 'refreshed' and does not ever fade.

Out in the Visual Field – Part Two

So much for all the wiring and processing that goes on in the visual pathway. What about the end product? It would seem only too obvious to say that the end product is what we see with our eyes - which is true. But what we see with our eyes (plural) is different from what we see with each eye (singular); for there is information about our surroundings that is only decodable from data obtained by both eyes working together, in what is called binocular vision. This can only be achieved if both eyes are situated relatively close together in the head and facing forwards, enabling them to focus on the same object at the same time. Some animals, though, for example, rabbits, have their eyes at the side of their head. Their main requirement, as potential prey, is to be able to see as far to the side and rear as possible so as to spot approaching predators early. Predators (and that includes us), need to be able to judge the speed and distance of potential prey as accurately as possible, and this is one of the main benefits of having binocular vision.

Binocular vision works because each eye sees an object from a slightly different point of view from its fellow eye. It also means that each eye of a pair sees an object in a slightly different position relative to other objects. An easy way to illustrate this is to hold up a pencil at arm's length and line it up with a relatively distant object (say, a tree across the road). When looking with just the right eye the pen will suddenly appear to the left of the tree, and vice versa for the left eye. The brain is able to compute all this information about position and movement to provide a proper three-dimensional picture of the world around us. Film-makers essentially use a technique of shooting with two cameras mounted a short distance apart to produce 3D films. The glasses one wears to view these films ensure that only the appropriate image is seen by each eye and the brain, making the computations as described above, converts these into a (virtual) three-dimensional picture. To appreciate how important binocular vision is for locating accurately objects in the environment, just try catching a ball with only one eye open. It's harder than you'd think.

To be accurate, there are some cues about distance and position available from the picture formed by one eye, such as the fact that nearer objects tend to appear larger and more distinct than distant objects; and our knowledge of perspective, ie the way parallel lines converge to a common distant vanishing point. It is this class of cues that artists employ in order to create a realistic three-dimensional picture on a two-dimensional surface.

For good binocular vision to develop in children, it is vital that both eyes have reasonably good, roughly equal vision, and that they are well co-ordinated in their movements. Early examination in order to discover an eye with poor vision or a 'turn' (squint) is very important in this respect. As we saw in Chapter One, the early years are critical for the development of vision, and that includes binocular vision.

Mapping the Visual Field

Apart from some schoolteachers who claim to have eyes in the back of their heads, it is pretty obvious that we cannot see behind us. But how far from the straight ahead does our visual field extend? Figures vary but, generally, the visual field of each eye extends around 65 degrees upwards, 75 degrees downwards, 60 degrees inwards (nasally) and 100 degrees outwards. Approximately the inner third of the eyes' visual fields overlap, and this is the area of binocular vision.

As we have seen, the nerve fibre wiring all the way from the retina to the visual cortex is very precisely arranged. This means that the representation of each part of the retina (and therefore the visual field) can be associated with particular sites at each part of the visual pathway. Now suppose we could create a map of an individual's visual field: if there is a piece missing from the field of one or both eyes, we could work out where in the visual pathway is the problem that has caused the visual defect. Remember that the visual pathway meanders past many important structures in the brain, so if one of those structures is damaged it is likely also to damage the visual pathway at that point. Imagine the enormous potential that exists for pinpointing damage within the brain merely by mapping out the visual field, without the need for costly and time-consuming scans. This is precisely what happens every day in an optometrist's practice thanks to modern computerised equipment that can create a detailed visual field map in a matter of minutes. It is worth expanding on some of the types of visual field defects that can be mapped by these modern instruments, or *perimeters*, to illustrate just how useful a diagnostic tool visual screening is.

Put simply, a field defect in one eye only must place the problem in the optic nerve of that eye; between the start of the optic nerve at the eye (including the retinal fibres) and the chiasma, where nerve fibres cross over to join fibres from the other eye in the opposite pathway. Perhaps the most common of these defects is that found in glaucoma: the raised intraocular pressure initially damages discrete bundles of nerve fibres at the edge of the optic nerve head, and the resulting arc-shaped defect mirrors the path these fibres take as they fan out over a sector of the retina. Of course, glaucoma can affect both eyes, so defects eventually may be seen in both eyes.

The chiasma itself is sited in close proximity to the pituitary gland. A pituitary tumour pressing on the chiasma will damage the nasal nerve fibres from each eye as they cross over at this point, resulting in a characteristic field defect where the outside (temporal) half of both fields are affected. It is easy to appreciate that a person with this type of defect may well still feel that they can see clearly, while wondering why they are bruising both arms by constantly bumping in to things.

Once we are past the chiasma, damage to the optic tract anywhere in its path to the visual cortex in the occipital lobe of the brain will result in some form of defect of both the right or left halves of the eyes' visual fields. The right halves are affected by damage to the left optic tract, and vice versa. The approximate position of damage within the optic tract can be estimated by looking at the shape of the field defect, because the arrangement of bundles of nerve fibres varies along the tract. These types of defects are most commonly seen as a result of vascular accidents such as haemorrhages and aneurysms.

How is the mapping,or *perimetry*, of the visual field actually done? There are two methods of perimetry: static and kinetic. Static perimetry is perhaps the more commonly used in general optometric practice. It involves testing a whole range of points across the visual field. Basically, this is done by flashing a light briefly at each point and recording whether or not it is seen. A map is then plotted of any gaps in the visual field. But it is not an 'all or nothing' process. The lights can be presented at different levels of illumination so as to gauge the sensitivity of all parts of the field; one sector may be completely defective and insensitive to light, while a neighbouring sector may still register a bright light. The significance of this sort of finding is that it may indicate a dynamic situation where the field defect is expanding (from the insensitive to the partially-sensitive sector), which means that whatever is causing the defect is still actively changing.

Kinetic perimetry involves moving a target or light from outside the visual field to the point where it is first seen, and then bringing it all the way into the centre of the field to check for islands of field loss within the field's limits. This is repeated at many points around the whole field, to both create a contour of the extent of the visual field and to detect defects within the field. This can be quite a tiring exercise for the subject, but it can build up a very detailed picture – especially when the process is repeated with targets of different size, brightness or colour.

To re-emphasise the value of visual field screening, it is worth noting that the discovery of a visual field defect is sometimes the first sign of a significant cranial problem, discovered even before the patient is aware of any visual or other symptoms. It is yet another illustration of the eyes and visual system as an important indicator of general health.

We have now travelled from the front to the back of the eye and beyond. We have seen how the eye is a direct outpost of that most complicated and mysterious object, the brain. The senses of touch and hearing are essentially those of pressure detection. The senses of smell and taste detect chemicals. All those four senses have a limited range of distance within which they can detect a stimulus. The sense of sight is unique in relying on the detection of a quintessential, ubiquitous phenomenon of the universe, electromagnetic radiation. To be sure, human vision covers only a small part of the electromagnetic spectrum but the eye is far more versatile in the detection of electromagnetic radiation than any single measuring instrument of man-made construction.

The sense of sight gives us an amazing ability to navigate our environment and appreciate and understand the world around us. It enables us to communicate with our fellow human beings in much more complex ways than mere speech can, via the opportunity to interpret the subtleties of body language. It allows us a direct connection to the depths of space and time. Look up at the sky on a clear night. The light from many of the stars has taken many millions of years to travel across the universe.

Imagine a single photon setting out on its journey before the Earth was formed, before the oceans gave rise to the first living organisms, before primitive eyes evolved, before creatures crawled on to dry land, before the first sentient, self-aware animals evolved into the person reading these words; all that time the photon has been travelling across space at around 300,000 kilometres per second to enter your eye just as you look up in the sky, when it hits a retinal cell that sets off a cascade of chemical reactions that sends an electrical signal to your brain, that alerts you to the pinpoint of starlight out there. Other people may see that star too, but that photon has crossed interstellar space to reach your eye alone; it is your personal connection to the farthest reaches of the observable universe. Isn't the eye amazing?

WHO'S WHO IN OPTICS

The terminology surrounding the different branches of the optical profession can be quite confusing. Once upon a time there were 'oculists', who were usually medical practitioners, to look after the eyes, and 'opticians' who made lenses for spectacles and other optical instruments. And that was about it. Nowadays the provision of eyecare and optical correction is more fragmented, so the following list is aimed at clarifying the titles and roles of the different players in the optical game.

OPHTHALMOLOGIST

Ophthalmologists are medically-trained doctors who have undertaken further specialist training in treating eye disease (the traditional 'oculist'). They will usually be a fellow of the Royal College of Ophthalmologists, with the title Mr (or Miss, Mrs, Ms or other as appropriate) and letters FRCOphth after their name. An ophthalmologist who also lectures at a medical school may also attain the title of Professor. These are the people whose care you are under when referred to hospital with eye problems. Ophthalmologists will often have sub-specialties within the field of

193

ophthalmology; for example, cataract surgery, retinal disease, glaucoma, neuro-ophthalmology. To confuse matters, ophthalmologists may be known by the following descriptions (all of which can be preceeded by 'consultant'):

Eye specialist
Eye surgeon
Eye doctor
Ophthalmic surgeon

Sir Arthur Conan Doyle (1859 – 1930) was spectacularly unsuccessful in private practice as an ophthalmologist, a fact that persuaded him to concentrate on writing fiction.

OPTOMETRIST

Whether or not you recognise the term, an optometrist is almost certainly the person you go to see to have your eyes tested. Yet most people would still automatically say that they were 'going to the optician' for an eye test. After all, isn't it obvious that the optician tests your eyes, and who uses the word 'optometrist' anyway? In truth, we optometrists are as culpable as the general public in that if someone asks one of us what we do for a living, we're more than likely to give a little sigh inside and reply, 'I'm an optician' rather than use the optometrist word and get the inevitable response, 'What's that, then?' which necessitates an explanation that probably includes variants of the phrase, 'It's a sort of optician.'

So why 'optometrist' rather than 'optician'? Surprising though it may seem given the above discussion, the term 'optometrist' was adopted in this country in the late 1980s to avoid confusion. Up until then, practitioners were known as ophthalmic opticians but, in the eyes of the public, that title was often swallowed up within the more general term 'optician', of which there are several types. So, in 1987 the British College of Ophthalmic Opticians changed its name to the British College of Optometrists, borrowing the term used for the profession in the USA and several other countries. The word itself merely means 'vision measurer' which hardly does justice to the scope of the profession, but at least it is a protected title under the Opticians Act 1989 and is a recognisably distinct term within the field of optics.

Optometrists are not medically qualified, ie they are not doctors, and (with some exceptions, as described below) do not treat eye disease. But they are more than just 'vision measurers'. Optometrists are qualified to recognise eye disease and take the appropriate action, for example, to refer the patient to an ophthalmologist. They perform 'eye examinations' to determine the status of the visual system and correct, if necessary, any visual defects with spectacles or contact lenses. They can supply and fit these devices, although sometimes these functions are delegated to other professionals. In recent years, optometrists have begun to work more closely with ophthalmologists in schemes that delegate some ophthalmological functions to suitably-trained community practitioners. These might include monitoring diabetics for eye disease, providing fast-track referrals for cataract surgery or monitoring stable glaucoma patients.

Optometrists do not have the title 'Doctor' (unlike in the USA), although an optometrist may have earned that title through completion of a higher degree, say, a PhD in optometry. In 1995 the British College of Optometrists was granted a Royal Charter and changed its name to, simply, the College of Optometrists. As such, most optometrists will be members of the College and will have MCOptom after their name; a Fellowship is obtainable by examination, which entitles the use of FCOptom. Incidentally, one of the College's forerunners, the British Optical Association, founded in 1895, was the first professional body solely for ophthalmic opticians (as they then were) in the world, and the first to run professional examinations.

I have taken the liberty of going into more detail about optometrists partly because it my profession, but mainly because awareness of the title is still so vague even after over thirty years' usage in this country, not to mention knowledge of the breadth of an optometrist's work. One notable holder of the title is the Australian, Geoff Lawson, a hero from my student days, who managed to combine a career as an international cricketer with qualification as an optometrist. Finally, for handy summary:

Optometrist [modern name] = Ophthalmic optician [previous name]

DISPENSING OPTICIAN

Dispensing opticians do not perform eye examinations, but they are trained in all aspects of interpreting the resulting prescription with respect to the production of spectacles appropriate to the patient. They are expert in fitting, adjusting and modifying spectacle frames and have a wide knowledge of ophthalmic lenses. Although some optometrists do their own dispensing, many work in tandem with dispensing opticians, who will discuss with the patient their visual needs according to their lifestyle, and recommend suitable lens and frame types, along with relevant lens tints and coatings, to give the best visual and cosmetic results. Some dispensing opticians take a further diploma in contact lens fitting or low vision (the supply and fitting of aids for the visually impaired), enabling them to specialise in these areas. Qualification as a dispensing optician is via the Fellowship Diploma of the Association of British Dispensing Opticians, leading to the post-nominals FBDO.

ORTHOPTIST

The orthoptic profession is small and deals mainly with the diagnosis and management of disorders of binocular vision; conditions where the two eyes are not working together. Often this means children with a 'squint', or, 'turn' in the eye, but includes people with acquired double vision resulting from general, systemic, diseases such as diabetes, thyroid conditions or neurological disease. They

197

work in hospital eye departments as part of an ophthalmologist's team, and in recent years this has enabled them gradually to expand the scope of their work. Some optometrists are happy to manage squints in children but, if referred to hospital, it will be the orthoptist who looks after them.

MANUFACTURING OPTICIAN

These are the people who actually make the frames, spectacle lenses and contact lenses that you wear. Britain has a fine tradition in optical manufacturing, dating back at least to the late sixteenth century, when there was a boom in activity, particularly in the City of London. This lead to the formation of the Worshipful Company of Spectacle Makers (WCSM) in 1629, the sixtieth in order of precedence of the 110 Livery Companies (as of 2018), which aimed to impose quality control over the growing optical trade. For those who are interested there is a painting by Johann Zoffany of an optician in his workshop, which is in the Royal Collection and can be viewed on the Collection's website. The work, *John Cuff and His Assistant* (1772), depicts the eponymous subject - himself Master of the WCSM in 1748 - at his workbench (although it should be said that there is some controversy about the identity of the subject). The British optical industry still thrives, but it is now a truly global trade.

OPHTHALMIC MEDICAL PRACTITIONER (OMP)

There is a small group of around 600 medically qualified doctors who have passed a diploma or higher qualification of the Royal College of Ophthalmologists, who are then qualified to perform basically the same functions as an optometrist. It is possible, then, that if the person testing your eyes has the title 'Doctor', they may be an OMP rather than an optometrist with a PhD.

'THE OTHERS'

It would be remiss of me not to mention a very important 'behind the scenes' group of people, without whom a paper spectacle prescription would never be transformed into a physical pair of spectacles. These are the **optical technicians**, the craftsmen who take an order form from an optometrist or dispensing optician and cut and glaze the appropriate lenses into a frame. One can learn the rudiments of the craft on the job, but it takes a high degree of skill and technical knowledge to be proficient. These 'glazers' are in some ways the direct heirs of the seventeenth century opticians such as the aforementioned Cuff. Indeed, their qualifications are still administered by the WCSM. The highest level of qualification (the gold standard of the craft) entitles the holder to use the post-nominals SMC(Tech). As an aside, the famous Dutch philosopher Baruch Spinoza (1632 – 77) was an optical technician, or 'lens grinder', of notable quality. It is thought that long-term inhalation of glass dust contributed to his relatively early death.

There are other people you might meet in an optical practice, who might variously be styled **optical assistant**, **frame stylist**, **frame consultant** or **optical receptionist**. At one time these would all have been synonyms for a shop assistant with no formal optical qualifications and varying degrees of in-house training. The situation is changing. The traditional optical receptionist is, in my view anyway, one of the most important people in the practice, being, as they often are, the first point of contact for a patient. There is now a wide recognition for an enhanced role for so-called 'optical practice support staff'. The WCSM is at the forefront of this movement too, offering a range of courses and qualifications for such staff, including a new qualification equivalent to the SMC(Tech), namely the SMC(OA), where 'OA' stands for Optical Assistant. The goal of the WCSM is to provide dual manufacturing and retail pathways for non-professional staff to reach a high standard of practical knowledge and skill, preparing them, should they so desire, to continue on the career ladder to professional qualifications.

It is now possible to see a clear potential career path from optical support staff and optical technician to dispensing optician to optometrist and on to ophthalmologist. There are many people who have taken at least one of those steps. In some cases, the attainment of one qualification earns partial exemption from parts of the next qualification up. Probably the biggest step is from optometrist to ophthalmologist, as the optometrist has to begin by obtaining a medical degree before being then able to specialise in ophthalmology (although the optometry degree confers exemptions from some of the ophthalmology examinations).

This appendix is intended primarily, as its title says, as a guide to who's who in optics. But if it also reads as a sales pitch for a career in optics, that's great. Go for it, I say; it's a wonderfully interesting and diverse field of endeavour as, hopefully, this book has shown. There are so many levels to enter at – especially with the development of new optical apprenticeships - and so many opportunities for advancement. And if the preceding paragraphs also appear to be a long advertisement for the Worshipful Company of Spectacle Makers, then I must make a declaration: I am a Liveryman of the Company and can vouch for its educational and charitable work and for the fellowship it engenders among all branches of the optical world within a forward-looking organisation that nevertheless has its roots in the centuries-old traditions of London life.

MEASUREMENT OF EYESIGHT

Eyesight is generally measured by seeing how far one can read down a test chart comprising lines of letters of decreasing size. The letters need to be of standardised sizes and viewed at a common distance, otherwise the results would be fairly meaningless. But how were those standards arrived at? Why are the letters often viewed via looking in a mirror at the far end of a room? And what do the numbers that denote a level of vision mean?

To answer these questions, we must turn to the Dutch ophthalmologist, Herman Snellen (1834 – 1908). Based mainly at Utrecht, he made a huge contribution to his field, not least by inventing the eye test chart that bears his name and that you still read when you have an eye test. Test types for letter charts were already in use by Snellen's time, but his original idea was to standardise them to enable the vision test to be properly repeatable in any location.

Snellen's letters, which he called *optotypes*, were designed on a grid of 5x5 units. The letters themselves are of a size 5x5 units, while the thickness of all lines making up each letter is one unit. The letter design is *sans serif*, that is, entirely plain. Now follows an explanation of how Snellen chose his letter sizes: if geometry is not your thing (although it only concerns right-angled triangles), skip to the end of the next three paragraphs.

He defined the sizes of letters correlating with different levels of vision by making a triangle ABC and imagining letters standing vertically at different points along the line AB (see Figure 6 below). So a letter standing at BC is twice as tall as a letter standing half way along AB (matching the line DE). He chose a letter a tenth of the height of BC to represent normal vision when viewed at six metres, where the angle at A in the diagram is five minutes of arc (which is approximately 0.0833 degrees).

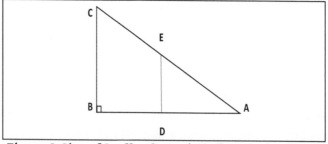

Figure 6. Size of Snellen letter is defined by its distance from angle A when forming the vertical side of a right-angled triangle (eg BC or DE).

Now he had standardised shapes and sizes of letters. His chart is designed to be viewed at a distance of six metres, far enough away for the eye's accommodation to be relaxed and so equating to distance vision. The letter at the top of his chart can be considered as the one of height BC. This letter, viewed from a distance of 6m, of a size that makes the common angle at A at a distance of 60m from A (ie when AB is 60m long), is given the notation 6/60. A letter about half way down the chart that makes the common angle A at 12m has the notation 6/12; and one near the bottom of the chart of a size that makes the common angle at A at 6m, has the notation 6/6 and is the 'normal' vision line referred to above.

In summary, the level of vision achieved on the Snellen test chart can be defined as follows:

<u>Testing distance</u>
Letter size

where testing distance is usually 6m. The top letter of the Snellen chart is 6/60 and the bottom line is usually 6/5. But what about the term '20/20 vision'? This derives from the American convention of working in units of feet; the equivalent distance in feet to 6m being 20ft. So having 20/20 vision is not perfect vision at all – equating to 6/6 vision, this is only the penultimate line on a standard Snellen chart.

We've now answered two of our three initial questions: how the standards for the letters on a test chart were arrived at and what the notation means. What about the mirror question? That's quite simple, really. Given that the accepted viewing distance of the chart is six metres, using a mirror on the opposite wall is merely a space-saving device. It means that the consulting room has only to be three metres long instead of six metres since, optically, light travels three metres from the chart to the mirror and another three metres back to the patient's eye. It also explains why many charts make use only of those letters that look the same whether viewed directly or in a mirror (ie, are symmetrical around a vertical axis); it means that the chart is suitable for use in a standard three-metre consulting room or when viewed directly in a six-metre room.

Another question may have occurred to you: what if a person can't recognise or name the letters? Other versions of the Snellen test have been devised for just this situation. There are charts made up entirely of either the letter E or the letter C, with the letter appearing in four different orientations. The limbs of the E or the gap in the C can be pointing up, down, left or right. The person has either to point in the relevant direction or to hold a template of the letter and turn it the correct way. There are also children's charts of pictograms; the pictures of trains, boats, and so on all conform to overall Snellen dimensions, although the lines within them strictly do not. More commonly used for children are flip-books of letters or pictograms that are held up a page at a time to be seen by the child in the mirror, the child pointing to the same image on a sheet that he or she holds.

It is worth mentioning that there are now in use other versions of the Snellen chart and other methods of measuring vision. Many optometrists use a computerised screen (viewed directly or via a mirror). One advantage of these screens is that they put up randomised lines of letters, so that the same line of letters is never encountered twice. This avoids the possible 'learning effect' of using a single chart. Also used are projection screens, whereby a projector at the patient's end of a three-metre room projects letters on to a matt grey screen at the opposite wall.

Other systems of vision measurement are logMAR and contrast sensitivity. Briefly, the letter sizes on the logMAR chart are calculated on a logarithmic scale, so that each line of letters is smaller by the same amount as the previous one (the jumps in size on the Snellen chart vary from line to line). A value is also assigned to each letter on a line depending on how many letters are on that line, thereby taking account of a phenomenon called the 'crowding effect', in which the presence of adjacent letters can affect the ability to identify a specific letter. In this way a more accurate assessment of vision can be made.

Contrast sensitivity is also thought to give a better measure of vision than the Snellen test. Imagine the difference between a bold black letter on a white background and a light grey letter on the same background. In essence contrast sensitivity tests how faint a letter can be before it is no longer distinguishable by an individual. Both these tests have their merits and, from an academic point of view, probably give a better measure of vision than the Snellen test. But the Snellen test is so entrenched and universally used that it will probably be the method of choice for some time to come.

Finally, a note about terminology. I have been using the term 'vision' throughout. Clinically, 'vision' or 'unaided vision' refers to the result achieved with the naked eye. The measurement achieved with the aid of spectacles or contact lenses is properly called 'visual acuity' and is abbreviated to 'VA'.

A NOTE ON SPECTACLE PRESCRIPTIONS

The present situation in the UK is that a copy of a spectacle prescription must by law be given to a patient at the end of an eye examination. If spectacles are not required, then a statement to that effect should be issued. From experience, it seems that this piece of paper is often ignored, lost or not handed out in the first place. But when notice is taken of it, the few numbers and symbols it contains is a source of endless confusion – so it is worth giving a little consideration here to what it all means.

The first thing to note is that, where the prescription for each eye is written side by side, it is (or should be) the convention to write the prescription for the right eye on the left-hand side of the page. This is because it is the same way around that a practitioner sees a patient's eyes when looking at them. Of course, the prescription should label clearly which refers to right and left eyes respectively, but the intuitive thing for a layperson to do may be to assume that the left eye's details are written on *their* left side.

One more thing regarding left and right. Each eye's prescription may be labelled 'Right' and 'Left' or simply 'R' and 'L'. Occasionally one still sees the terms 'OD' and 'OS' instead. These are abbreviations for the Latin terms *oculus dexter* and *oculus sinister*, meaning 'right eye' and 'left eye' respectively.

There are seven terms that may appear on the prescription form, the first five of which are usually given a specific box or space for their values to be entered in, and these are described below in the order in which they are written down:

Sph (sphere): The amount of long- or short-sightedness present, preceded by a plus or minus sign respectively, and specified in increments of 0.25 dioptre strength. A plus sign indicates longsightedness (hypermetropia) and a minus sign, shortsightedness (myopia). If the amount is zero, it is written as 'Plano' or sometimes as the '∞' infinity symbol.

Cyl (cylinder): The amount of astigmatism (see Chapter Three), specified in increments of 0.25 dioptre strength. If there is no astigmatism present the box is left empty. There are two equally valid conventions: preceding the figure with a plus or minus sign. The more common convention nowadays, for technical reasons to do with the methods used in determining the final prescription, is to use the minus sign convention. Note that the same prescription written in 'plus cyl' form will show a different value for both sphere and axis.

Axis: This specifies the orientation of the astigmatism. If an astigmatic eye is shaped like a lemon as opposed to an orange-shaped spherical eye, one can imagine the lemon lying on its side, standing on its end or at any angle in between. The axis stipulates where in that range of attitudes the curves that make up the 'lemon-ness' of the cornea stand. The axis is given as a number (in degrees) between zero and 180, but in fact zero is never used – 180 is always used to specify the horizontal (and 90 is vertical). If there is a cyl in the prescription, there will *always* be an accompanying axis. Likewise, if there is no cyl, the axis box will also be empty. By convention the degree symbol is never used: this is to avoid confusion of the type where 10 degrees might be mistaken for 100 if the degree symbol were written too large.

Prism: As discussed briefly in Chapter Nine a prism is an element sometimes added to a prescription to aid the two eyes in working together where there is some muscular deficit or misalignment. It does not affect the focusing power of the lens. The units of prism seen in a spectacle prescription are mostly small numbers in the range 1-4, although they may be higher and may be specified in steps of ½ or ¼ of a unit. The number is sometimes accompanied by a small triangle, the symbol of prism units.

Base: This specifies the orientation of a prism. A prism has a profile of an isosceles triangle: two equal-length sides and a base. The direction the prism needs to be oriented in a spectacle lens depends on the direction of weakness or misalignment of the eyes' muscles and is almost always specified by one of four positions of the prism base: Up, Down, Left, Right. The exceptions relate to rare combinations of muscle imbalance that I will not go into here, apart from mentioning that one does sometimes see two prism values given for an eye each with their own associated base, one of which will be horizontal (In, Out) and one vertical (Up, Down).

Add: Prescription forms all have spaces to enter Distance and Near (or Reading) prescriptions. As a Near prescription is determined basically by adding more power to the Distance sphere, a shortcut for writing out both prescriptions in full is to give the Distance prescription and then the amount added on for Near, that is, the Add (short for 'addition'). By definition, this always has a plus sign. Note that while most commonly the Add is the same for both eyes, it is not necessarily so. A further shorthand occasionally seen is to have the Add written only once, with the suffix 'OU', these letters being the abbreviation for the Latin, *oculus uterque*, meaning 'both eyes'.

BVD (Back vertex distance): This does not form part of the prescription proper, so there is not usually a specific space for it on the prescription form. In simple terms the BVD refers to the distance between the back surface of the lens and the front surface of the eye and is given in millimetres. It specifies the test conditions that resulted in the given prescription and is an indication that the spectacles should be fitted at a similar distance. This is important for stronger prescriptions because the higher the power of a lens, the more its effective optical power changes with distance from the eye. So, it is considered good practice to in-

212

clude this measurement on prescriptions with a sphere of more than, say, 5-6 dioptres.

ACKNOWLEDGEMENTS

I would like to thank Mr John Shilling, retired oph-thalmologist at St Thomas' and Past Master of the Worshipful Company of Spectacle Makers, for taking the trouble to read through a draft of this book, for making some eminently sensible suggestions for imrovements and pointing out errors of fact. It goes without saying that any errors that remain are mine alone.

Thanks also to Bob Hutchinson, President of the Royal Society of Medicine GP with Primary Healthcare Section, for his practical advice and assistance in various ways.

Last but not least, thank you to my wife, Julie, who has, in so many ways that I can't even begin to list, enabled me to get this book written.

INDEX

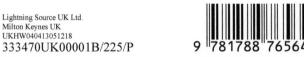